MW01234545

HYPNOSIS AND GUIDED MEDITATIONS FOR WEIGHT LOSS AND ANXIETY

2 BOOKS IN 1

REWIRE YOUR BRAIN TO STOP EMOTIONAL EATING, LOSE WEIGHT FAST AND FEEL AMAZING.

MANAGE YOUR EMOTIONS, REDUCE STRESS, STOP WORRYING AND OVERTHINKING.

Awakening Transformation Academy

BOOK 1
GUIDED MEDITATIONS FOR WEIGHT LOSS

BOOK 2
GUIDED MEDITATIONS FOR ANXIETY

GUIDED MEDITATIONS FOR WEIGHT LOSS

POWERFUL MEDITATION

AND HYPNOSIS PROGRAM

TO REWIRE YOUR BRAIN, STOP EMOTIONAL EATING

AND LOSE WEIGHT FAST.

BURN FAT, INCREASE YOUR SELF-ESTEEM

AND FEEL AMAZING!

Awakening Transformation Academy

Table of Contents

Introduction

One of the hardest parts about losing weight is having to wait so long to see the results. While there isn't a way to lose 20 pounds overnight, you can reshape your mentality so that you can grow your patience for the process. When you fully recognize time and how that plays into weight loss, you won't be looking at the scale every hour, begging for results. Instead, you will be happy with your journey and able to recognize the incredible way that your body is changing. This is a visualization exercise that is going to help you get in the right mindset to lose weight fast.

This meditation is going to be a visualization. You are going to want to make sure that you are in a comfortable place where you can drift off and go to sleep if you want to. We are going to take you through the scene that will await you at the end of your natural weight loss journey. We often have many ideas of what we want to get from our weight loss process, but we don't always visualize what the actual setting could be. In this meditation, we are going to help you understand the realistic scenario that you could find yourself in after you've managed to lose the weight. Close your eyes and keep your body as relaxed as possible. Start to focus on your breathing. Breathe in through your nose and out through your mouth. Concentrate the air as it travels through your body so that you will be able to shut out any negative or toxic thoughts more easily than you have in this moment.

Chapter 1
What Is Hypnosis For Weight Loss?

This hypnosis program is for people who want to lose weight, feel confident about their bodies, get toned and be healthy.

If you're reading this right now, one thing is for certain and that is that you want to make some serious changes to your body. As a woman, your self-confidence and self-esteem is highly influenced by how you feel about the current state of your body. Make no mistake about it, when you wake up and don't like the appearance staring back at you in the mirror, it sets the whole tone for the rest of the day – negative, for the most part.

You know very well that when you feel great in your own skin, your day just moves along better. You've put your heart into trying to achieve a body that you can feel good about, but alas, not much has come from your efforts. All of this is about to change.

This hypnosis program will help you to:

- Stay committed into trying to achieve a body that you have been searching for all this time.

- Naturally burn up more calories on a day to day basis doing nothing.

- Set up a proper plan that is going to work with your body and help you release fat storage from all the trouble spots on your body.

The book includes:

Hypnosis for naturally losing weight: The hypnosis will help you to change your negative mental views and turn them into positive ones, practice gratitude for weight loss, visualize, accept and appreciate your fabulous healthy body. It will emphasize on how to set and focus on your goals to keep that negativity at bay since losing weight needs consistent reminders and focus on proper mental preparations. Always keep yourself motivated and train yourself to think positive all the time.

Meditation for relaxation: A meditation to reduce muscle tension, lower blood pressure, calm the mind, eliminate stress and achieve mental and physical condition. You can practice it into your everyday life to help you deal with stress, relax and have peace of mind. Deep rest and relaxation achieved through meditation is therefore great for rejuvenating the body to leave you well and mentally serene.

Positive affirmations for weight loss: You will find a sequence of powerful affirmations for weight loss which are intended to magnify your focus on the positive reality you desire and the possibility thereof. They will help you take control of your motivation and release doubt, giving you the power to pave the steps in front of you, as you stride confidently toward your manifesting goals. You are now striding confidently toward manifesting your weight loss goals!

Well, you had better accept it if you want to see optimal results. But as a woman, you need to be on top of your game. To get the most out of the program you need to choose one of the aforementioned hypnosis and focus on it. Once you have finished this program, you should then feel ready and confident to put your best foot forward and see the optimal results that you are looking for.

Dieting plans using to these restrictions can definitely work, but only in the short run. In spite of avoiding regaining those lost pounds, there is a better way to choose.

With the right approach, you get to satisfy your sugar cravings, you get to enjoy some of your favorite foods and you still get to reach your optimal weight.

It should be noted that there are many weight gain triggers other than food. For instance, living in a stressful environment or not getting enough sleep can affect your waistline.

Accordingly, in spite of losing weight and keeping it that way, you need to work on your weight gain triggers just as you need to work on your meal plans.

Moreover, you need to work on changing your weight loss mindset, you need to rewire your thoughts about fitness and healthy living in the in order to stay on the right track in the long run.

Making the decision to lose weight was easy because everyone wants to look good. However, to enjoy success in the long run, you need dedication and commitment to truly follow through on your decision.

This is when things become more difficult as following your decisions over some time can be daunting. This is the main reason why people tend to quit.

For the sake of avoiding this happening to you, in addition to working on slightly changing your dieting pattern, you also need to embrace simple, easy-to-follow, yet effective weight loss tips which will keep you focused and motivated.

Moreover, losing weight is not only about looking good, but way beyond this. Losing weight can benefit you in numerous ways and your dieting choices can definitely make a difference both in the present and in the future.

The best way to go is to follow a dieting plan you can make work in the long run. Once there, with simple weight loss tips you get to stay on the right track, you get to keep your motivation and you get to work on your fitness and weight loss mindset.

These, when combined, lead you towards a healthy lifestyle you have always wanted to embrace, but you have lacked motivation, inspiration or knowledge.

In the direction of starting the journey on the right foot, it is important you understand why you gain or lose weight, what different weight gain factors are and other scientific facts revolving around shedding and gaining pounds.

Why Is It Hard To Lose Weight

You can say goodbye to obsessing over your daily calorie intake, over obsessing over how many carbs you ingested today.

You can say goodbye to extremely restrictive bans on foods as well as on other forced behaviors in pursuance of focusing on getting back into shape in a healthy, natural way by following your body's biology.

You have probably blamed yourself, or your lack of self-discipline in the past. You probably have blamed calories and your dieting formulas which most certainly did not bring anything good your way.

The truth is that there is no one and nothing to blame here. Every step you have taken in the past can teach you something which will help you to succeed in the future.

Another truth is that losing weight can be an extremely difficult thing to do and there are several different reasons behind this.

If you are focused on the weight loss industry, you have probably been told many times before how easy it is to shed those additional pounds.

The industry generally suggests you take this pill, drink that beverage or buy this equipment and simply enjoy your additional pounds melting on their own.

The truth is that the industry generates billions of dollars every year thanks to individuals who spend their money on different weight loss tools and products which can only be effective in the short-run.

Accordingly, many people struggling with weight are still overweight despite hundreds of dollars spent in the industry.

Now, you probably wonder why it is so hard and challenging to lose those additional pounds. It should be noted that there is no magical pill, magical tool or magical equipment that can make the process runs smoothly.

Dieting plans which suggest you completely change your dieting pattern, quit eating your favorite foods and similar restrictions do not work.

There is also scientific evidence as clear as it can get that suggests that cutting your daily calorie intake will not by any means lead to health gains or long-term weight loss.

It would be logical that most dieters have realized they have wrong dieting patterns, but still, individuals set those same weight goals every year.

The truth is that dieting failures are the norm. There is also a massive stigma surrounding heavier people and on many occasions, we can witness the massive blame game which is directed towards dieters who are not able to shed those additional pounds.

On the other hand, looking from a scientific point of view, it is clear that dieting most certainly sets up a truly unfair fight.

Many people are confused to learn that dieting plans suggesting extreme dieting changes, but that this only comes as a result of the statements does not square with their previous observations.

There are some thin people who consume junk food and still stay thin without their food choices affecting their weight.

These people most usually think that they stay in shape due to their dieting habits, but the truth is that genetics plays a massive role in helping them stay fit.

These people are praised over their dieting choices as others can only see what they consume, but they cannot examine what is inside their genes.

The Importance Of Genetics

Due to the role of genetics, many individuals struggling with excess pounds will not be as thin as other people even if they embrace the same dieting choices as them and consume them in the exact same quantities.

The bodies of those heavier people can run on fewer calories than thin people require which may sound like a promising thing.

On the other hand, this means that they have more calories left, stored as fat in the body after eating the same food in the same quantities as thinner people.

This means that they need to consume fewer foods than thin people in order to shed pounds. Once they have followed some dieting plan for some time, their overall metabolic state changes which means that they need to consume even fewer calories in pursuance of losing further weight.

It isn't only genetics which makes thin people stay thin, but it is also their mindset revolving around dieting and fitness.

For thin people, as they are non-dieters, it is very easy to ignore those sugary treats and desserts which for heavier people seem like a massive challenge and obstacle on their weight loss journey.

For heavier people, these treats and sugary candies seem as if they are almost jumping around cheerfully making them approach and eat them.

This being said, dieting of any kind causes specific neurological changes which make people more likely to be focused on foods and notice foods everywhere.

Once they notice foods, those neurological changes happening in the brain are what makes it almost impossible to not think about food.

Thin people more often than not forget about those sweet treats on the desk, but dieters tend to keep obsessing over them.

As a matter of fact, dieters seem to crave these foods even more due to those neurological changes.

Moreover, these neurological changes make food taste better due to the fact they cause a greater rush of dopamine or the reward hormone.

This is the exact same hormone releases when drug addicts or substance abusers use their drug. Individuals who are non-dieters do not suffer from these kinds of rushes, so they can peacefully leave a piece of cake untouched.

Dieters also tend to struggle with another issue revolving around neurological changes which affect their hormonal balance.

They face another uphill battle when their leptin hormone or satiety hormone levels go down. Due to this hormonal change, dieters require even more foods to consume in pursuance of feeling full.

This means that they felt hungry following their dieting plans and over some time they feel even hungrier once again due to hormonal changes.

Weight Stigma

Individuals usually see thin people and are impressed by their self-discipline, self-determination or their willpower and self-control.

Yet, should it be considered great self-control or great willpower to avoid consuming foods, when you are actually not hungry.

It really is a true willpower or true self-control when you are able to avoid eating foods you do not notice at all and you do not get any reward rush out of it.

The plain truth is that anyone would be able to resist sugary sweets or any food under these specific circumstances, as there is no need for any willpower or great self-control to avoid foods when you are not actually hungry and when you have no rushes to worry about.

Even though thin people do not need any extra self-control or willpower in these cases, if they do need it, their self-control and willpower would function optimally due to the fact that they are non-dieters.

On top of these extreme circumstances, dieters who need to struggle with dieting of any kind also disrupt their cognition which is especially effective over their executive function.

The executive function is a process which promotes and helps with self-control. Hence, people following strict dieting plans have less self-control and willpower in those situations when they need more willpower.

On the other hand, in the same situations during which dieters struggle, non-dieters have plenty of self-control and willpower even though they do not need it.

And there is also another fact, if thin people were to eat delicious cakes, treats, and other tempting foods, their metabolism burns more calories by far when compared with the dieter's metabolism state.

All of this means that thin people are mistakenly given some credit for staying fit and in shape at this job that comes easier to them than for those individuals following some dieting plan.

These facts lead to the very cruel irony which makes it very hard to keep losing weight for individuals who have been following some dieting plan.

Yes, it is physically possible to lose weight in the long-run, but just a small minority of dieters actually manages to keep losing weight for months or years.

Following the trend, this battle does not come without demoralization, stigma, and damages to their mindset which dieting does to their physiology both in the short-run and in the long-run.

It is very easy to see why the majority of dieters regain the weight they have lost.

No matter the obstacles and challenges, we have to work on changing the stigma surrounding weight, especially weight gain.

You struggling with additional pounds does not make you weak in any way. The factors affecting weight gain and weight regain and they have nothing do to with your dieting choices.

Hence, be impressed by every single step you take, be grateful for every small goal you reach and remind yourself that you are not weak, but you are a victim of a very unfair battle.

This battle is won by only a few who are more focused on staying healthy than losing weight, who are determined to improve their weight not by any artificial means, but only in a natural way.

The Impact of Weight Stigma

The main question here is whether anti-obesity and anti-overweight attitudes are the ones contributing to these outcomes in obese and overweight individuals.

First, we need to clarify this term of weight stigma. It is stereotyping or discrimination towards individuals based on their weight. Weight stigma is also known as weight-based discrimination or weight bias.

One of the major health risks of weight stigma lies in the fact that it can lead to extremely increased body dissatisfaction which is one of the leading factors contributing to the development of various kinds of eating disorders.

When it comes to the best-known factor leading to the development of an eating disorder, it is definitely the very common and highly present idealization of being thin as seen in media as well as other social-cultural environments.

However, it is never acceptable by any means to discriminate against someone based on any physical features and weight is one of them.

On the other hand, weight stigma which includes blaming, shaming and concern trolling individuals who struggle with their weight happens more commonly than we want to admit.

The fact is it happens everywhere, at home, at school, at work and in some cases even in the doctor's office.

This tells us that weight discrimination is more prevalent then we think and according to the latest studies on the topic, it even occurs more often than age or gender discrimination.

Another truth is that weight stigma is very dangerous increasing the risk for different behavioral and psychological issues such as binge eating, poor body image, and depression.

In fact, weight stigma has been documented as one of the risks for low self-esteem, depression and extreme body dissatisfaction.

Moreover, those individuals who struggle with weight stigma also tend to engage more often in binge eating.

They are also at a significantly increased risk for developing some type of eating disorder and they are more likely to be diagnosed for BED or binge eating disorder.

Those individuals struggling with weight stigma also generally report that their family members, friends, and their physicians are the most common sources of their weight stigma struggles.

When it comes to family members and friends, diet talk and weight-based teasing are more often than not related to extreme weight control patterns, unhealthy behaviors, and weight gain as well as binge eating.

This being said, weight stigma in health care is yet another very important concern showing the magnitude of this problem.

The topic which show health care professionals and providers, when talking to overweight and obese patients tend to provide them with not valuable health information, tend to spend not enough time with them and tend to see them as annoying, and undisciplined as well as uncompliant with their weight loss treatment.

There is also a massive issue regarding popular obesity and overweight prevention campaigns. Attention given to weight control and obesity definitely has skyrocketed in the past several years.

By doing so, the industry has ingrained words such as diet, obesity epidemic and BMI into our regular vocabulary.

Chapter 2
Meditation Program For Weight Loss

What is meditation?

Meditation comes from the word "medicina", which is a Latin word and originally means natural medicine. Meditation signifies that we do not identify our thoughts with the voice and emotions in our heads, but go beyond them and notice them objectively without negative or positive judgments. This technique can be practiced even while cleaning, and we don't need specific circumstances to meditate. If we do something from the heart, we can say that we are meditating. Meditation is the art of entirely redirecting focus to only one thing.

Meditation is a changed state of awareness that cannot be produced by will or forced. In this regard, it is similar to sleep, because the more we want to sleep, the more alert we will be. Meditation usually refers to a state of mind whereby the body is consciously carefree and relaxed, and our spirit is let go of peace and concentration within ourselves. Meditation does not merely imply sitting or lying down for five to ten minutes in silence. Meditation indeed demands mindful work. The mind must be relaxed and balanced. At the same time, the brain must be alert so that it does not allow any disturbing thoughts or desires to penetrate. We begin meditation with our effort. Still, when we delve intensely into ourselves, we see that it is not our individual self that allows us to enter the state of meditation. The

Supreme or Creator meditates within and through us, with our deliberate attention and permission.

The aim is to seek peace and freedom from disturbing thoughts. In such cases, the meditator achieves an escape from the environment so that from a psychological point of view, the experience could even be called a changed state of consciousness. When we can make our minds calm and still, we will touch a new existence awakened within us. If our mind is discharged and tranquil, and our entire being becomes an empty vessel, then our internal presence can call upon eternal peace, light, and mercy to flow into and fill this vessel. This happens during meditation.

The effect of meditation

Meditation has been used in many cultures for thousands of years because of its numerous benefits: it reduces anxiety, and makes people feel happy. In the short term, meditation has mainly psychological advantages, but in the long run, it has physical outcomes. Those who try meditation can enjoy its benefits in the short term such as balance, greater peace and vitality, and a decreased need for sleep. Physical effects can be experienced in just a few months: among other things, blood pressure may return to normal, or digestion may improve. So you can imagine how beneficial it can be in the long run.

The University of California's Neuroscience Laboratory has been researching the impacts of meditation on the brain's structure for years. Their most recent research has studied long-term effects in the minds of habitual meditators compared to non-meditators. According to their results, the cerebral cortex of long-term meditators is more marked than that of non-meditators, indicating increased cognitive performance. The Frontiers in Human Neuroscience published research which became a milestone in science because it has long been believed that the brain mass reaches its peak in the early twenties, and then begins to narrow slowly (Bae, Hur, Hwang, Jung, Kang, Kim, Kwak, Kwon, Lee, Lim, Cho, & Park, 2019). Previously it was a widespread opinion that there was no way to interrupt this process. However, it is now known that the brain retains its plasticity to some extent, and it can physically change as a result of meditation. Earlier studies have shown that for long-time meditators, both gray matter and white matter in the brain have increased in weight. (The former contains the cells of the brain nerve cells; the latter contains the neuronal cell-forming projections). The number of neurons in the cortex changes only very rarely in adulthood. One group of the current research involved 28 men and 22 women, their average age was 51, and they had all been meditating for an average of 20 years. The oldest participant was 71, and the most experienced meditator had been practicing daily for 46 years. The researchers performed MRI scans of participants' brains and compared them to 50 non-meditating members of the control group.

Regular practice can increase the advantages of meditation. According to research, the more practitioners repeated deep breathing techniques and other meditation methods, the more they relieved the symptoms of arthritis, reduced their pain, increased their immune systems, manifested healthier hormone levels, and lowered blood pressure. According to the researchers, this explains that a person's mental state can change his physical condition and gives an added motivation to why traditional Tibetan, Indian, and

Ayurvedic medicine view meditation and the repetition of mantras as therapeutic.

Hundreds of scientific documents confirm the positive healing and health benefits of meditation. Here are some of them.

During the first twenty minutes of meditation, metabolism is reduced by sixteen percent. The body deeply calms down during transcendental meditation, which is the result of decreased cellular oxygen utilization due to reduced metabolism. It also decreases heart rate and stabilizes blood circulation (Dillbeck, & Orne-Johnson, 1987). Besides, the blood pressure decreases, and muscular tension and anxiety consequently disappear. Meditation has proven to be effective in overcoming chronic anxiety and in increasing self-esteem (Eppley, Abrams, & Shear, 1989). Meditation is also an effective way to create relaxation and reduce physiological stimulation. The essence of the phenomenon is a decrease in respiratory rate, oxygen consumption and carbon dioxide exhalation. Breathing is not only rarer but more profound, vital capacity increases from resting 450-550 ml to 800-1300 ml (up to 2000 ml for some master meditators) and remains consistent throughout. However, a lower respiratory rate is not offset by deeper breathing, resulting in a 20% reduction in respiratory volume under rest.

Several sports psychologists think that meditation may be appropriate for improving athletic performance (Syer, & Conolly, 1984). Meditation can help lessen the stress of competition, but with some practice, an athlete can also learn how to relax different muscle groups individually and detect complex differences in muscle tension.

Throughout meditation, the athlete can anticipate the next event (such as skiing downhill) in such detail that the visualization of the action can be almost perfectly synchronized with the action itself. The skier anticipates how he will start from the starting position, gliding down and accelerating, avoiding the gates, and doing the entire race in his head. By framing images of successful performance, an athlete may attempt to program their muscles and body for the best results.

The power of meditation

Meditation has impressive power because we associate emotions coming from the depths of the soul with conscious thought. In meditation, the individual is brought into the same frequency as the origin of the Inner Self, that is, the Universe itself, and thus is directly connected to the consciousness sphere of the Universe. In this state, there is no time limit, so the visualized fulfillment can immediately expand to the physical level. As a result of regular meditation, we obtain numerous benefits in a physical and mental sense. We will be healthier because when we focus on our breathing, our blood pressure drops, our heart rate slows down; consequently, we become calmer. It helps us have a clearer mind, sort out our thoughts and emotions, making our communication more productive both at work and in social life. We can focus more easily and accordingly feel less stressed. We become more aware of our emotions; hence, we can manage them more effectively. We find a solution sooner in areas of our lives where we feel stuck. It promotes the processing of mental problems. It helps to find peace and balance. We get closer to understanding ourselves, the people around us, our lives, and our mission.

When we accept ourselves as we are, we become positive, joyful, and attractive. This will make our existing relationship more intimate or, if we are alone, the desired partner will come into our lives.

What is a guided meditation?

Unlike the traditional type, guided meditation is aimed at a specific purpose, and for beginners, it is one of the best ways to approach this practice. It is also called guided visualization. In this type of meditation, you form mental images of places or situations where you can feel relaxed. Most of the time, this is practiced with a teacher's help or a leader who is not necessarily present in the room where the meditation occurs. It's enough to include listening to a recording and meditating on it.

Guided meditations are not all the same: it depends on the purpose you want to achieve through this practice. Do you just want to relax? Fight insomnia? Become more resilient? Accept a major change? Lose weight?

In most guided meditations, it's essential to try to use as many senses as you can: the smells, the lights, the sounds, the textures. Usually guided meditations have a musical background that invites the mind and body to relax: sounds of nature such as rain, rainforest, sea waves or the sound of a waterfall; or more traditional music like that of the Native American characterized by the sound of flutes, tubes and rattles. Choose the musical background you prefer, what is important is to create the best condition to relax. To start, you can do a very quick guided meditation for beginners. The basic principle is to pay attention to what you do, always keep it in mind from the beginning to the end of the practice. Close your eyes and start taking three deep breaths, inhaling through your nose and exhaling from your mouth. When you breathe in you are full of positive energy and when you exhale all kinds of negative energies, such as stress, tension and worries, abandon you. Find your breath and feel your body. Simply observe it (Headspace, n. d.).

Chapter 3
Guided Meditation For Weight Loss

Meditation exercise 1: Release of bad habits

Sit comfortably. Relax your muscles, close your eyes. Breathe in and breathe out. Do not cross your feet because this will lock you away from the desired experience. Hold your hands together to connect your logical brain hemisphere with your instinct.

Concentrate on your back now and notice how you feel in the bed or chair you are sitting in. Take a deep breath and let your stress leave your body. Now focus on your neck. Observe how your neck is joined to your shoulders. Lift your shoulders slowly. Breathe in slowly and release it. Feel how your shoulders loosen. Lift your shoulders again a little bit then let them relax. Observe how your neck muscles are tensing and how much pressure it has. Breathe in and breathe out slowly. Release the pressure in your neck and notice how the stress is leaving your body. Repeat the whole exercise from the beginning. Observe your back. Notice all the stress and let it go with a profound breath. Focus on your shoulders and neck again. Lift up your shoulders and hold it for some moments, then release your shoulders again and let all the stress go away. Sense how the stress is going away. Now, focus your attention to your back. Feel how comfortable it is. Focus on your whole body. While breathing in, let relaxation come, and while you are breathing out, let frustration leave your body. Notice how much you are relaxed.

Concentrate on your inner self. Breathe slowly in and release it. Calm your mind. Observe your thoughts. Don't go with them because your aim is to observe them and not to be involved. It's time to let go of your overweight self that you are not feeling good about. It's like your body is wearing a bigger, heavier top at this point in your life. Imagine stepping out of it and laying it on an imaginary chair facing you. Now tell yourself to let go of these old, established eating and behavioral patterns. Imagine that all your old, fixed patterns and all the obstacles that prevent you from achieving your desired weight are exiting your body, soul, and spirit with each breath. Know that your soul is perfect as it is, and all you want is for everything that pulls away to leave. With every breath, let your old beliefs go, as you are creating more and more space for something new. After spending a few minutes with this, imagine that every time you breathe in, you are inhaling prana, the life energy of the universe, shining in gold. In this life force you will find everything you need and desire: a healthy, muscular body, a self that loves itself in all circumstances, a hand that puts enough nutritious food on the table, a strong voice to say no to sabotaging your diet, a head that can say no to those who are trying to distract you from your ideas and goals. With each breath, you absorb these positive images and emotions.

See in front of you exactly what your life would be like if you got everything you wanted. Release your old self and start becoming your new self. Gradually restore your breathing to regular breathing. Feel the solid ground beneath you, open your eyes, and return to your everyday state of consciousness.

Meditation exercise 2: Forgiving yourself

Sit comfortably. Do not cross your feet because this will lock you away from the desired experience. Hold your hands together to connect your logical brain hemisphere with your instinct. Relax your muscles, close your eyes.

Imagine a staircase in front of you! Descend it, counting down from ten to one.

You reached and found a door at the bottom of the stairs. Open the door. There is a meadow in front of us. Let's see if it has grass, if so, if it has flowers, what color, whether there is a bush or tree, and describe what you see in the distance.

Find the path covered with white stones and start walking on it.

Feel the power of the Earth flowing through your soles, the breeze stroking your skin, the warmth of the sun radiating toward you. Feel the harmony of the elements and your state of well-being.

From the left side, you hear the rattle of the stream. Walk down to the shore. This water of life comes from the throne of God. Take it with your palms and drink three sips and notice how it tastes. If you want, you can wash yourself in it. Keep walking. Feel the power of the Earth flowing through your soles, the breeze stroking your skin, the warmth of the sun radiating toward you. Feel the harmony of the elements and your state of well being. In the distance, you see an ancient tree with many branches. This is the Tree of Life. Take a leaf from it, chew it, and note its taste. You continue walking along the white gravel path. Feel the power of the Earth flowing through your soles, the breeze stroking your skin, the warmth of the sun radiating toward you. Feel the harmony of the elements and your state of well being. You have arrived at the Lake of Conscience, no one in this lake sinks. Rest on the water and think that all the emotions and thoughts you no longer need (anger, fear, horror, hopelessness, pain, sorrow, anxiety, annoyance, self-blame, superiority, self-pity, and guilt) pass through your skin and you purify them by the magical power of water. And you see that the water around you is full of gray and black globules that are slowly recovering the turquoise-green color of the water. You think once again of all the emotions and thoughts you no longer need (anger, fear, horror, hopelessness, pain, sorrow, anxiety, annoyance, self-blame, superiority, self-pity, guilt) and they pass through your skin and you purify them by the magical power of water. You see that the water around you is full of gray and black globules that are slowly obscuring the turquoise-green color of the water. And once again, think of all the emotions and thoughts you no longer need (anger, fear, horror, hopelessness, pain, sorrow, anxiety, annoyance, self-blame, superiority, self-pity, guilt) as they pass through your skin, you purify them by the magical power of water. And you once again see that the water around you is full of gray and black globules that are slowly obscuring the turquoise-green color of the water.

You feel the power of the water, the power of the Earth, the breeze of your skin, the radiance of the sun warming you, the harmony of the elements, the feeling of well-being.

You ask your magical horse to come for you. You love your horse, you pamper it, and let it caress you too. You bounce on its back and head to God's Grad. In the air, you fly together, become one being. You have arrived. Ask your horse to wait.

You grow wings, and you fly toward the Trinity. You bow your head and apologize for all the sins you have committed against your body. You apologize for all the sins you have committed against your soul. You apologize for all the sins you committed against your spirit. You wait for the angels to give you the gifts that help you. If you can't see yourself receive one, it means you don't need one yet. If you did, open it and look inside. Give thanks that you could be here. Get back on your horse and fly back to the meadow. Find the white gravel path and head back down to the door to your stairs. Look at the grass in the meadow. Notice if there are any flowers. If so, describe the colors, any bush or tree, and whatever you see in the distance. Feel the power of the Earth flowing through your soles, the breeze stroking your skin, the warmth of the sun radiating toward you. Feel the harmony of the elements and your state of wellbeing. You arrive at the door, open it, and head up the stairs. Count from one to ten. You are back, move your fingers slowly, open your eyes.

Chapter 4
Meditation For A Mindfulness Diet

One of the best ways to transition into a diet that's centered around weight loss is to do so using mindful eating. All too often, we eat well beyond what is needed, and this may lead to unwanted weight gain down the line.

Mindful eating is important because it will help you appreciate food more. Rather than eating large portions just to feel full, you will work on savoring every bite.

This will be helpful for those people who want to fast but need to do something to increase their willpower when they are elongating the periods in between their mealtimes. It will also be very helpful for the individuals who struggle with binge eating.

Portion control alone can be enough for some people to see the physical results of their weight-loss plan. Do your best to incorporate mindful eating practices in your daily life so that you can control how much you are eating.

This meditation is going to be specific for eating an apple. You can practice mindful eating without meditation by sharing meals with others or sitting alone with nothing but a nice view out the window. This meditation will still guide you so that you understand the kinds of thoughts that will be helpful while staying mindful during your meals.

Mindful Eating Meditation

You are now sitting down, completely relaxed. Find a comfortable spot where you can keep your feet on the ground and put as little strain throughout your body as possible. You are focused on breathing in as deeply as you can.

Close your eyes as we take you through this meditation. If you want to actually eat an apple as we go through this, that is great. Alternatively it can simply be an exercise that you can use to envision yourself eating an apple.

Let's start with a breathing exercise. Take your hand and make a fist. Point out your thumb and your pink. Now, place your right pinky on your left nostril. Breathe in through your right nostril.

Now, take your thumb and place it on your right nostril. Release your pink and breathe out through your nostrils. This is a great breathing exercise that will help to keep you focused.

While you continue to do this, breathe in for one, two, three, four, and five. Breathe out for six, seven, eight, nine, and 10. Breathe in for one, two, three, four, and five. Breathe out for six, seven, eight, nine, and 10.

You can place your hand back down but ensure that you are keeping up with this breathing pattern to regulate the air inside your body. It will allow you to remain focused and centered now.

Close your eyes and let yourself to become more relaxed. Breathe in and then out.

In front of you, there is an apple and a glass of water. The apple has been perfectly sliced already because you want to be able to eat the fruit with ease. You do not need to cut it every time, but it is nice to change up the form and texture of the apple before eating it.

Breathe in for one, two, three, four, and five. Breathe out for six, seven, eight, nine, and 10.

Now, you reach for the water and take a sip. You do not chug the water as it makes it hard for your body to process the liquid easily. You are sipping the water, taking in everything about it. You are made up of water, so you need to constantly replenish yourself with nature's nectar.

You are still focused on breathing and becoming more relaxed. Then, you reach for a slice of apple and slowly place it in your mouth. You let it sit there for a moment and then you take a bite.

It crunches between your teeth, the texture satisfying your craving. It is amazing that this apple came from nature. It always surprises you how delicious and sweet something that comes straight from the earth can be.

You chew the apple slowly, breaking it down as much as you can. You know how important it is for your food to be broken down as much as possible so that you can digest it. This will help your body absorb as many vitamins and minerals as possible.

This bit is making you feel healthy. Each time you take another bite, it fills you more and more with the good things that your body needs. Each time you take a bite, you are making a decision in favor of your health. Each time you swallow a piece of the apple, you are becoming more centered on feeling and looking even better.

You are taking a break from eating now. You do not need to eat this apple fast. You know that it is more important to take your time.

Look down at the apple now. It has an attractive skin on the outside. You wouldn't think by looking at it about what this sweet fruit might look like inside. Its skin was built to protect it. Its skin keeps everything good inside.

The inside is white, fresh, and very juicy. Think of all this apple could have been used for. Sauce, juice, and pie. There are so many options when it comes to what this apple may have become. Instead, it is going directly into your body. It is going to provide you with the delicious fruit that can give you nourishment.

You reach for your glass of water and take a long drink. It is still okay to take big drinks. However, you are focused now on going back to small sips. You take a drink and allow the water to move through your mouth. You use this water not just to fill your body but to clean it. Water washes over you, and you can use it in your mouth to wash things out as well.

You swallow your water and feel it as it begins to travel through your body. You place the water down now and reach for another apple slice.

You take a bite, feeling the apple crunch between your teeth once again. You feel this apple slice travel from your mouth throughout the rest of your body. Your body is going to work to break down every part of the apple and use it for nourishment. Your body knows how to take the good things that you are feeding it and use that for something good. Your body is smart. Your body is strong. Your body understands what needs to be done to become as healthy as possible.

GUIDED MEDITATIONS FOR WEIGHT LOSS

You are eating until you are full. You do not need to eat any more than what is necessary to keep your body healthy. You are only eating things that are good for it.

You continue to drink water. You feel how it awakens you. You are like a plant that starts to sag once you don't have enough water. You are energized, hydrated, and filled with everything needed to live a happy and healthy life.

You are still focused on your breathing. We will now end the meditation, and you can move onto either finishing the apple or doing something relaxing.

You are centered on your health. You are keeping track of your breathing. You feel the air come into your body. You also feel it as it leaves. When we reach zero, you will be out of the meditation.

Twenty, 19, 18, 17, 16, 15, 14, 13, 12, 11, 10, nine, eight, seven, six, five, four, three, two, one.

Chapter 5
Meditation To Burn Fat

Our bodies were designed to burn fat. It is the way that they provide the body with energy when we haven't given it enough through the foods we eat. We require more energy when we workout, so our bodies will burn more fat during these processes.

Though it can sound so simple on paper, it will be rather challenging to always include these things in our lives. This meditation is going to help guide you through the journey of getting the body you want, with a visualization exercise to help you see your goals laid out clearly. Listen to this first when you are in a relaxed position in case you become calm to the point of sleep.

After you know how you react, you might include this when you are doing yoga or another form of light exercise to help keep you grounded and relaxed.

Fat Burn Meditation

Narrator: This is a visualization meditation. I am going to take you on a mindfulness journey through your body. To start, ensure that you are somewhere that you can be fully relaxed. You don't want to have any distractions around, and the only thing that you are going to focus on now is the air that is coming in and out of your body.

Narrator pauses for 3 seconds

Narrator: Let your mind go blank. As thoughts begin to creep in, gently push them out with each exhale. Focus on nothing else other than the air that enters your body, and how it exits.

Narrator pauses for 3 seconds, breathing in and out

Narrator: When we count down from ten, you are going to imagine that you are in the middle of the woods. There is a light trail and you are walking down it.

Breathe in for one, two, three...

And out for three, two, one...

You will be in the woods in ten, nine, eight, seven, six, five, four, three, two, and one.

Narrator pauses for 3 seconds

Narrator: You are walking through the woods, noticing everything that surrounds you. There are trees, birds, and even a little stream that you can hear the water running from.

You are feeling incredibly good in this moment, healthy and focused. You haven't eaten in a little bit, but you aren't very hungry just yet. You felt your stomach grumble, but it was just a small signal that you need to eat. Nothing is causing you pain or discomfort. You are focused on right now only, and nothing else.

You are walking up a hill now, a slight incline. You feel the burn start to occur in your legs. As you continue to walk, you begin to realize that your body is starting to burn fat.

You don't have to tell your body to do this. You don't have to take a pill to do this. Your body knows how to do it on its own.

You supply it with healthy food that doesn't add as many calories as you need for energy to your body, meaning that you are burning fat faster.

You put it through workouts in order to burn fat. The combination of both of these are helping you to lose weight.

Narrator pauses for 3 seconds

Narrator: You won't notice in the mirror immediately after burning the fat, but you are feeling it immediately in the way your body functions. Each time your stomach growls, you feel it. Every time you take a step, you feel it. As your body is continuing to get stronger and stronger, and push you closer and closer to the goals that you want, you feel lighter and lighter.

Your body is burning more and more fat. You are becoming more and more relaxed, focusing only on your breathing and the good feeling circulating through your entire body. The only thing that you concern yourself with is shedding the pounds.

Narrator pauses for 3 seconds

Narrator: You are only burning fat. You aren't doing anything to add fat, which means that your body's only option is to use what is already there as an energy source.

You consistently make choices to burn the fat from your body. You are always looking for ways to become lighter and lighter. You feel as your waist is getting slimmer and slimmer.

It feels good to drop the weight. It feels amazing to finally let go of all that has been holding you back.

The more weight that you are burning, the easier it is to lose even more. There is nothing that is going to keep you from getting the things that you want in this life. You are working with your body to get the things that you have been hoping for.

Narrator pauses for 3 seconds

Narrator: You continue to walk through the woods with the realization that you are a part of nature just like all that surrounds you. Your body was made in order to keep you as healthy as possible. Now, it is time to train your brain so that it is optimized for health as well.

Your brain will try to do what it thinks is right for your health. It wants you to eat ice cream, so you feel better right now. It wants you to sit on the couch instead of workout so that you can save your energy. Your body is only thinking of the "now."

You are training your brain to think about the future. You are accepting all that surrounds you, and that you are a part of this nature just as the rest. You are connected to the earth and feel the natural processes flow through your body. You are highly aware of all of the things that you need to do in order to keep your body as healthy as possible.

Narrator pauses for 3 seconds

Narrator: Your body feels better and better the further that you walk. Sometimes you feel a slight strain in your legs, but nothing that is painful. It is simply your body doing its best to burn as much fat as possible. It is your body working hard. It is a good pain, one that makes you feel healthier, stronger.

You have water with you that you take a drink of. This is the fuel that helps to keep your body going. You provide it with everything necessary in order to continually work hard.

Your body will always burn fat. It is designed to use what you already have stored within you. Each time you make a healthy choice, it makes you feel healthier.

Every time you do something good for your body, you are burning fat. You continue to burn fat, always feeling lighter and lighter.

Narrator pauses for 3 seconds

Narrator: You are more relaxed now. Your mind understands what it needs to do to be healthy. You are starting to feel lighter every day.

The forest around you is fading.

As we come to the end of the meditation, remember to focus on your breathing. You will either be able to drift off to sleep or move onto other meditations needed for weight loss mindset.

As we reach ten, come out of the forest and back into reality where you will be focused only on burning fat and losing weight.

Narrator counts to ten

Chapter 6
Heal Your Relation With Food

All too often, we eat well beyond what is needed, and this may lead to unwanted weight gain down the line.

Mindful eating is important because it will help you appreciate food more. Rather than eating large portions just to feel full, you will work on savoring every bite.

This will be helpful for those people who want to fast but need to do something to increase their willpower when they are elongating the periods in between their mealtimes. It will also be very helpful for the individuals who struggle with binge eating.

Portion control alone can be enough for some people to see the physical results of their weight-loss plan. Do your best to incorporate mindful eating practices in your daily life so that you can control how much you are eating.

This meditation is going to be specific for eating an apple. You can practice mindful eating without meditation by sharing meals with others or sitting alone with nothing but a nice view out the window. This meditation will still guide you so that you understand the kinds of thoughts that will be helpful while staying mindful during your meals.

Mindful Eating Meditation

You are now sitting down, completely relaxed. Find a comfortable spot where you can keep your feet on the ground and put as little strain throughout your body as possible. You are focused on breathing in as deeply as you can.

Close your eyes as we take you through this meditation. If you want to actually eat an apple as we go through this, that is great. Alternatively it can simply be an exercise that you can use to envision yourself eating an apple.

Let's start with a breathing exercise. Take your hand and make a fist. Point out your thumb and your pink. Now, place your right pinky on your left nostril. Breathe in through your right nostril.

Now, take your thumb and place it on your right nostril. Release your pink and breathe out through your nostrils. This is a great breathing exercise that will help to keep you focused.

While you continue to do this, breathe in for one, two, three, four, and five. Breathe out for six, seven, eight, nine, and 10. Breathe in for one, two, three, four, and five. Breathe out for six, seven, eight, nine, and 10.

You can place your hand back down but ensure that you are keeping up with this breathing pattern to regulate the air inside your body. It will allow you to remain focused and centered now.

Close your eyes and let yourself to become more relaxed. Breathe in and then out.

In front of you, there is an apple and a glass of water. The apple has been perfectly sliced already because you want to be able to eat the fruit with ease. You do not need to cut it every time, but it is nice to change up the form and texture of the apple before eating it.

Breathe in for one, two, three, four, and five. Breathe out for six, seven, eight, nine, and 10.

Now, you reach for the water and take a sip. You do not chug the water as it makes it hard for your body to process the liquid easily. You are sipping the water, taking in everything about it. You are made up of water, so you need to constantly replenish yourself with nature's nectar.

You are still focused on breathing and becoming more relaxed. Then, you reach for a slice of apple and slowly place it in your mouth. You let it sit there for a moment and then you take a bite.

It crunches between your teeth, the texture satisfying your craving. It is amazing that this apple came from nature. It always surprises you how delicious and sweet something that comes straight from the earth can be.

You chew the apple slowly, breaking it down as much as you can. You know how important it is for your food to be broken down as much as possible so that you can digest it. This will help your body absorb as many vitamins and minerals as possible.

This bit is making you feel healthy. Each time you take another bite, it fills you more and more with the good things that your body needs. Each time you take a bite, you are making a decision in favor of your health. Each time you swallow a piece of the apple, you are becoming more centered on feeling and looking even better.

You are taking a break from eating now. You do not need to eat this apple fast. You know that it is more important to take your time.

Look down at the apple now. It has an attractive skin on the outside. You wouldn't think by looking at it about what this sweet fruit might look like inside. Its skin was built to protect it. Its skin keeps everything good inside.

The inside is white, fresh, and very juicy. Think of all this apple could have been used for. Sauce, juice, and pie. Instead, it is going directly into your body. It is going to provide you with the delicious fruit that can give you nourishment.

You reach for your glass of water and take a long drink. It is still okay to take big drinks. However, you are focused now on going back to small sips. You take a drink and allow the water to move through your mouth. You use this water not just to fill your body but to clean it. Water washes over you, and you can use it in your mouth to wash things out as well.

You swallow your water and feel it as it begins to travel through your body. You place the water down now and reach for another apple slice.

You take a bite, feeling the apple crunch between your teeth once again. You feel this apple slice travel from your mouth throughout the rest of your body. Your body is going to work to break down every part of the apple and use it for nourishment. Your body knows how to take the good things that you are feeding it and use that for something good. Your body is smart. Your body is strong. Your body understands what needs to be done to become as healthy as possible.

You are eating until you are full. You do not need to eat any more than what is necessary to keep your body healthy. You are only eating things that are good for it.

You continue to drink water. You feel how it awakens you.

You are like a plant that starts to sag once you don't have enough water. You are energized, hydrated, and filled with everything needed to live a happy and healthy life.

You are still focused on your breathing. We will now end the meditation, and you can move onto either finishing the apple or doing something relaxing.

You are centered on your health. You are keeping track of your breathing. You feel the air come into your body. You also feel it as it leaves. When we reach zero, you will be out of the meditation.

Twenty, 19, 18, 17, 16, 15, 14, 13, 12, 11, 10, nine, eight, seven, six, five, four, three, two, one.

As mentioned previously, you should work and invest time and effort into reaching your desired body weight, not because of some thin body ideal circling around and not because of other people around you, but because weight gain in addition to helping you be more satisfied with your body image also brings numerous health benefits which are crucial on top of all other weight loss effects on your life.

The truth is that you do not have to lose some excess amount of weight to experience weight loss health benefits as losing only several pounds can make a huge difference.

For instance, losing ten pounds for a person weighing two hundred pounds improves her overall health state, make her feel better, more energized and much more.

Losing only ten pounds can rapidly ease up on your joints, remove some pressure off your knees as well as remove pressure off your other lower body joints which can wear out easily when you have to carry around those additional pounds.

Additional fat accumulated in the body can also cause various types of chronic inflammatory disorders as chemicals contained in the body, which tend to do tissue damage while damaging your joints as well.

Therefore, losing weight can prevent this from happening as well as reduce your risk for developing arthritis at some point later in life due to your weight.

Losing those extra pounds also can decrease your chances of developing some types of cancers. In fact, there is one study showing that a female who lost at least five percent of her body weight lowered her chances for developing breast cancer by twelve percent.

There is no clear proof that losing weight can protect you from other types of cancer, but even the slightest weight loss progress decreases the chances of developing breast cancer.

For instance, overweight females who lose extra pounds also tend to lower their hormone levels which are linked to the development of cancer cells including androgens, insulin, and estrogens.

If you are more likely to develop type 2 diabetes, weight loss is absolutely your way to go to delay or even prevent it from occurring.

Moreover, in addition to losing weight in these cases, moderate exercise for at least thirty minutes per day is also highly recommended.

On the other hand, if you have already been diagnosed with diabetes, losing those additional pounds can help you in many different ways such as keeping your blood sugar levels in control, lowering your odds of the condition causing some other health issues and lowering your need for taking all of those medications.

By losing additional pounds, you can also lower your levels of bad LDL cholesterol just by embracing healthy dieting options.

Unlike balancing those LDL cholesterol levels, balancing those levels of good HDL cholesterol is harder, but not impossible by losing body fat and by exercising regularly.

Just as you can balance your cholesterol levels, by losing those additional pounds, you can also bring down your triglyceride levels which are responsible for transporting energy and fat storage throughout the body.

High triglyceride levels mean you are more likely to have a stroke or heart attack, so moving closer to those healthy triglyceride levels is crucial for maintaining an optimal health state.

Those who are overweight and struggle with high blood pressure can absolutely make a huge change by losing those additional pounds.

As you know, having excess body weight puts the body under more stress so the blood starts pushing harder against the artery walls.

In these cases, the heart needs to work harder as well. In order to avoid suffering complications related to high blood pressure, trimming only five percent of your total body mass can make a massive change.

Another dieting tip for lowering high blood pressure includes eating plenty of low-fat dairy products, plenty of foods and veggies and cutting down on salty foods.

Individuals who struggle with excessive weight are at much greater risk for developing sleep apnea due to the excess fat situated in their throat tissue.

When the body relaxes when sleeping, that throat tissue can slightly drop down blocking the airway which can make people stop breathing periodically over the night.

Fortunately, shedding only several pounds of your overall body mass is in some cases enough to prevent sleep apnea and avoid the health issues which it brings.

Body fat accumulated on the abdomen or belly area tends to give off damaging chemicals which interfere with insulin effects which balance blood sugar levels.

Despite the fact that the pancreas works harder in order to produce more insulin, blood sugar levels can still go up. Fortunately, losing excess weight even only several pounds can prevent or reverse this from occurring.

There are numerous studies conducted on the topic which suggest that losing weight brings good night sleep which is less possible when you are overweight or obese.

Losing excess weight also leads to better mood as it may surely chase away your blues.

Moreover, weight loss will also make you feel better and more satisfied with yourself bringing a better body image and improved sleeping pattern due to weight loss may be one of the reasons.

There is also one study conducted on the topic showing that depressed individuals who are also overweight felt much better after losing an average of eight percent of their body weight.

The same study also suggests that they will feel even better if they keep losing weight in the future.

Shedding additional pounds also brings down various types of inflammation. Fat cells which are located on the abdominal area, in some cases, release damaging chemicals which inflame and irritate tissues throughout the body.

This is connected to various health issues such as heart attack, arthritis, stroke, and heart disease.

Fortunately, moving towards your optimal weight can easily lower the amount of those damaging chemicals in the body reducing the chances of developing these illnesses.

There are also some lifestyle benefits which weight loss brings such as greater self-esteem, improved energy and focus, decreased stress, improved mood, and improved vitality as well as greatly improved body image.

Weight loss also brings several social benefits as well such as greater motivation to stick to your exercise program or to your dieting program.

There are some individuals reporting that weight loss improved their mood and decreased stress also improved their personal relationships with family members and friends.

Changing Your Mindset

The very first step you need to take on your weight loss journey requires you to change your weight loss mindset. This is the first as well as the most important step for sustainable weight loss.

As you work on changing your weight loss mindset, you, in fact, rewire what you actually think about weight loss, so your overall weight loss journey can serve you better.

In other words, you need to cultivate your own weight loss state of mind. This psychological change you need to embrace can be even more challenging than adding a few additional greens to your plate.

This is something which needs to be done. First of all, keep in mind that there are three words you should ban from your mind as you embark on this journey.

These words are "I do not", "will not" and "cannot." These are three short words you need to ban in order to succeed as they just come from your mind and have nothing to do with your inner strength or with what you can achieve.

If you use them often, they can have a massive indirect impact on your weight-loss journey as well as on your fitness level.

Therefore, you need to flip the entire script and leave that negative talk behind. Individuals who are trying to lose weight commonly say do not simply due to their negative past experiences.

For instance, someone saying I do not like veggies simply reminds herself of those old experiences which do not have anything to do with her current behavior.

For this reason, your old experiences should not dictate your present behavior. If there are some I cannot or I do not terms in your vocabulary, you need to flip the script and turn them into I do and I can.

This will motivate and encourage you to move further and

after several days you will be able to pick your new pace with ease.

If your current fitness level is low, your "I cannot" words may be blocking your success. Instead of saying I cannot do ten push-ups, say I will try and I will succeed. You need to try as it is better to try and fail than fail to try.

You can start with two push-ups and every new day you add one more push-up, so you move further until you reach your fitness goal.

Your weight loss journey must start with you changing your mindset and rewiring what you think about weight loss.

There are numerous physical ways for overcoming your weight loss plateau such as changing your dieting habits and embracing physical activity.

Nonetheless, without changing your mindset, these tricks will only work in the short-run providing no sustainable weight loss journey as there is always some underlying thought keeping you from sustainable weight loss.

Unless you go out there and address it, you will keep struggling on the road. For instance, many females tend to lose pounds as soon as they start making healthier dieting choices, but their weight loss progress tends to stop before they are completely satisfied with what they see in the mirror.

The truth is that losing weight in a sustainable way is much more than shedding those additional pounds which seem to be melting away at the very beginning of the journey.

The trick is to keep losing weight after that initial period. Many females fail in this step as after periods of losing weight, their progress simply freezes.

The main reason for this happening is that very common weight loss plateau present keeping you from losing weight in the long run.

In order to overcome this issue, there is no any magic trick you can do except changing your weight loss mindset.

Chapter 7
Meditation For Weight Loss

There are various meditation techniques to lose weight because there are various ways to meditate. In this practice, breathing is fundamental as it is for our life. In some techniques it only consists of controlling well the way of breathing.

There are meditation exercises to lose weight, which greatly reduce anxiety since in many cases it is one of the main causes of a person having a hard time losing weight.

There are many meditation techniques that will help you lose weight because there are various ways of meditating and in this case breathing is essential.

The best meditation weight loss techniques:

1) Pratyahara

Pratyahara is a technique in which the negative information entering the mind is reduced and the positive information is increased.

When you spend too much time around a negative person, for example, who pressures you and makes you eat emotionally, you can isolate yourself from this adult, which helps to reduce emotional eating.

Alternatively, if you find yourself inspired by some of your friends and you want to lose weight, you can start hanging around more with those friends, which will increase your weight loss motivation.

Pratyahara is a mechanism where negativity is minimized and positivity is enhanced. Look at the above connection.

Applied to get in shape, that simply means you take in more positive information and experiences to help support your weight loss journey and take in less information that keeps you from getting in shape.

2. Mindfulness

Mindfulness is about understanding what's happening in your mind.

Most people are not aware of their thinking, which is why they are so greatly affected by their feelings.

They think, for example, "I need to eat chocolate," and go and get chocolate automatically.

A careful approach would be to say, "Alright, that's just a chocolate feeling, just an idea, it's not real, I don't really need candy in my head." Distancing yourself from your cravings in this way gives you power over them. It helps you avoid the cravings.

Instructions You'll need 1 piece of comfort food / junk food you'll still consume for this workout. Your pick.

Go in a quiet and peaceful place.

Place the junk food in front of you a few feet on the table / board.

Using good posture to sit comfortably.

Relax for two minutes Train your attention on the fact that your breath will come and go through the gap between your nose and mouth.

Take 25 attentive breaths.

Mind your dream junk food (the one before you).

Focus your mind on this food's effect in your head (don't look at the food itself, center on the food's mental impression).

You will find that certain feelings emerge when you concentrate your attention on the meal. You're going to have specific food ideas. The detrimental interaction with food is created by these emotions. We need these feelings to get rid of.

Each time you feel Each thought, SEE the thinking to get rid of the feelings (imagine that you are staring at yourself as if you were spectating yourself). First, tell yourself, "It's just an idea. At last, imagine blowing the idea away from you until it disappears completely.

Take the food.

You will experience different emotions again while holding the food in your mouth.

Take a minute to see the kinds of thoughts you're going through.

Tell yourself again that they're just thoughts. They're not facts in your head, they're just fantasies.

Now, I'm going to use the analogy of a chocolate bar to continue this workout, but you can start with whatever food you have.

Remove the bar of chocolate. Thought about it. Focus your mind on the flavor, colors, scent, sound, and any other part of the food 100 percent.

Notice again the kinds of thoughts that you are experiencing. Speak to yourself, "It's just feelings. They're not reality. "Imagine the thoughts floating in the distance.

Slowly eat the food. Bite into it, catch it and quit in your mouth. Don't go drinking. Think of the taste.

Stay mindful of your emotions with the food in your mouth. Speak to yourself, "It's just feelings. They're not true. "Imagine the thoughts in the distance floating away.

Swallow. Swallow.

Start until there's no food left.

You're shifting your thoughts and feelings about food with the weight loss meditation technique above.

This helps eliminate the negative thoughts about food that you have.

This method helps the subconscious to get rid of your food-related negative and illogical thoughts and feelings. In other words, you tell the mind that food is not pleasure, enjoyable, comfort, or anything else. Nutrition is nourishment.

You may have been a little shocked when you did the exercise above when I instructed you to delete ALL ideas, even good thoughts, during the exercise. At one point you might have thought (for example) "Food is nutrition. I will sleep right. "That's a good idea, isn't it? And why do you get rid of it?

The explanation to get rid of all emotions and not just the bad ones is that thoughts live as a matrix of our head. Thoughts are like a string fragment that is really poorly twisted. It doesn't necessarily lead to another good thought to consider one good thought. If you say "I'm going to eat well," your next idea is just as likely to be "No I'm probably not going to eat because I have a bad diet" as it is "Yeah, I'm going to eat healthy and exercise."

This is a simple exercise that will change the way you feel about your favorite food completely. It will change your mindset to junk food absolutely. And it will greatly reduce your cravings and make your diet better.

3. Visualization Meditations For Weight Loss

Visualizations are methods of therapy including visualization and visual imagery. You construct a mental picture of who you really want to be when you do a visualization meditation. Then you meditate on this image, which makes you feel that you can achieve your goal. It greatly increases the fitness drive and weight loss.

Try this method. "Sit quietly and concentrate on your breath for a few minutes. That's going to help you relax.

Now imagine the whole body as you would like it to be. What are you going to look like? What are you going to feel like? What's special about you? Imagine the specifics of these things now tell yourself how you're going to get there. Which moves do you take to get in shape?

Now see the steps above until you reach the ideal type of body.

4. Mind Body Meditation For Weight Loss

This method increases the connection between your mind and body, improving your self-control. It's a technique for changed body scanning.

1. Lie down with a good posture or sit down.

2. Close your eyes and focus on breathing. Fill your nose with 10 deep breaths.

3. We're going to guide the body's consciousness. This will increase the connection between mind and body. Start at your bottom. Just be aware of your feet. Concentrate on them. Observe and sound in or out of your feet. Explore the emotions there. Touch your feet (mentally).

4. Now move your body up systematically. Shift from your knees to your calves to your lower legs to your upper legs to your pelvis to your chest to your arms, wrists, back to your shoulders, to your body, chin, and finally head.

5. Sometimes you will feel discomfort in your body parts. Imagine breathing warm air in that area asking your body to relax if this is the case. This is going to ease the stress.

6. Now be mindful of the whole body and the emotions that run through you. This will increase your sensitivity. You will be more conscious of the sensation that precipitates the hunger the next time you experience a desire for food. That knowledge is going to give you more self-control.

7. Meditation for Weight Loss Visualization (Dhyana Meditation Technique) This is a very powerful meditation technique for weight loss. It's going to help you lose weight and keep your diet alive.

You must create a very convincing mental image of a better you in this diagram.

You'll see yourself as all you want to be. You must prepare your mind to know what you really want.

This will turbo-charge the loss of weight.

1. Use good posture to sit comfortably. Make sure that your body is aligned correctly.

2. Close your eyes and concentrate a few minutes on breathing. Breathe, breathe.

3. That's the fun bit. You will create a mental picture of yourself regularly as the person you really want to be. And you don't want to part from me. I want you to be absolutely amazing to see yourself. I want the same thing you want to be your own. It's all right. You're ready?

4. Start with the nose. What would look like your face? See that. See that. See your lovely skin. Notice how the wrinkles are zero. You look pretty. Consider that in detail.

5. The upper portion of your body. You might want a six pack if you're a male. You may want a lean and sleek look if you're a kid. Dream that your upper body is perfect.

6. Tone of the legs? Smooth? How are you going to want them? Picture that in depth.

7. Everything else: fill in your ideal body with any other info.

8. Imagine that this perfect thing you're doing with weight loss is incredible. You are doing something that you can only do once you have been able to lose weight. Maybe you've just run a marathon. Maybe you're on a stage with people watching you. Whatever it is that you like, imagine it in depth.

9. Bring it all together so you can picture something spectacular accomplishing your best self.

10. Affirmation: after accomplishing this amazing thing, what would your ideal self say? Choose an affirmation and imagine in your mind saying it LOUD.

11. Imagining the ideal self in depth is important. You really need to see that perfect body and really imagine getting that amazing thing done and really hear the positive affirmation in your head.

Using Meditation For Weight Loss When Depressed Most people who overeat do so because they have a negative food relationship. Maybe the best example of this is eating comforting people.

Nutrition is not just protein for comfort eaters, it is a method of protection that they use when they feel depressed or anxious. They feel stressed, they want something beautiful, they eat some delicious food, they feel better. But then, for eating too much, they feel bad. It makes them mindful of their diet. We felt stressed and depressed afterwards. So they're eating something good again and the vicious cycle begins anew.

A relaxed eating person correlates diet with sadness, pain, and relaxing. Food is what they are going to do when they feel depressed. This provides healing for them. It's all a habit in thought.

The same applies to people who, for other reasons, overeat.

Many people associate a luxurious lifestyle with good food. They want the luxury lifestyle to eat lots of food.

Others associate food with socialization.

None of these are safe connections.

Meat is nourishment, nothing.

The key to have a healthy food partnership is to remove the illogical food thoughts and beliefs and see that food is just protein. Live, not for any other reason, to nourish the body.

The perfect body and mind you're after can be accomplished. The meditation techniques for weight loss that we have looked at will help.

Enlightened people like you and I know the loss of weight occurs in the head.

The power of the subconscious to resist cravings, to inspire us to lose weight, and to help us through stressful times... these talents are worth much more than anything you can get at the gym.

The best way of thinking produces the right body.

Chapter 8
Portion Control Hypnosis
(Go In-Depth And Very Accurate)

It can be tempting to give into the promises we see from celebrities and other big brand ads about losing weight. They make it seem so effortless and fun, but when we start the journey ourselves, we soon discover that it is not so simple. This hypnosis is a process that will aide in your weight loss journey and provide for you a natural way to shed the pounds.

You will be guided through the process of feeling better, mindful eating, goal-oriented thoughts, and dedication to the body. This hypnosis is a little different than others and will involve "I" statements. Allow these thoughts to come into your brain as if they were your own.

Natural Weight Loss Hypnosis

Narrator: First you will need to find a calm and quiet place with little distraction. Lay down flat on the ground or bed, or sit with your legs crossed and back comfortably straight, your palms face up and resting on your knees. Once you are in this position begin taking long deep breaths from the stomach, in through the nose, and out the mouth.

Narrator breathes with listener for 5 seconds

Narrator: Good. As you breathe focus in on each of your

muscles, letting them constrict and then retract. Move on to the next one. Constrict, retract. Once all of your muscles are relaxed and your mind has focused on your inner and outer breaths, you'll want to clear your mind of all distractions. Imagine as you exhale, all the worries in your life leave with that one outward breath. Continue this until your mind is completely clear and your breath naturally falls into a rhythm.

Narrator pauses for 3-5 seconds

Narrator: As you continue to focus on these breaths, listen to the words carefully, repeat them in your head if you need to. These are affirmations that will change the way your mind thinks about weight loss and a healthier you. I do not need to participate in any diet plan. I do not need to sign up for one specific workout. I am able to go through with the weight loss all on my own. I am capable and ready to lose the weight naturally, using my own body to do this.

Narrator pauses for 3 seconds

Narrator: My body was designed to keep me as healthy as possible. The first step is deciding that I want to lose weight. This is a step that I have already agreed to. I have continually wanted to lose weight and have this be a part of my lifestyle.

Narrator pauses for 3 seconds

Narrator: I am devoted to making the best decision possible for my health. I am learning self-control and focusing on knowing what the best thing for my body is going to be. I understand when I should say "no," and when I need to push myself through something that might be a bit more challenging. I have recognized what bad habits I have done in the past, and I have created new habits that I can start to add to my future.

Narrator pauses for 3 seconds

Narrator: I understand why I need to lose the weight. I am no longer doing this just for looking good. I am doing this because I need to be healthier. I want to feel good all the time. I want to be able to have confidence and love myself easier.

Narrator pauses for 3 seconds

Narrator: I recognize that I need to love myself in this present moment. I cannot do this journey if I do not believe in myself. I am my own trainer. I am the person that is going to be encouraging me more than anyone else. I am the one who is going to be holding all of the power over my life for the rest of my time on this Earth. I am the one who needs to remember the things that are most important for achieving my dreams.

Narrator pauses for 3 seconds

Narrator: I love myself more than I ever have, which is why I am making this journey. If I do not learn to accept myself the way I am right now, then I will never fully be able to love the person that I am, even after I have made the transformation.

I am my own best friend. I have the ability to lose all of the weight that I want because it is part of who I am. It is natural for me to lose the weight the way that my body designed me to do so.

Narrator pauses for 3 seconds

Narrator: I am going to eat less calories than what I am used to eating right now. I am going to exercise more than what I am used to doing right now. I am going to do this so I can burn more calories and lose even more weight. I am dedicated to this lifestyle because I deserve it. I am focused on shedding the pounds because of all the various health benefits that come along with being more in shape.

Narrator pauses for 3 seconds

Narrator: I am going to eat foods that are healthy for me. I will not deprive myself of any nutrition. I will eat in moderation, but I will never starve myself. I will make sure to not overeat, but I will never completely keep food from my body.

I will exercise as often as I can. I will push myself on days that I feel like staying home instead, but I will never push myself to a point that I physically hurt myself. I will know when I need to try a little harder, and I will know when it is OK to lighten up.

Narrator pauses for 3 seconds

Narrator: I will learn all of these things through trusting my body. Not only do I have the natural processes to lose weight already inside of me, but I have what is needed to trust myself through my own intuition. I understand the importance of listening to my gut. I recognize how I can read what I need to do, and know what isn't necessary. *Narrator pauses for 3 seconds*

Narrator: I have made mistakes in the past, and there were moments where I didn't judge the situation properly. I will always know how to best listen to my voice as I continue to move forward in this life. I will only grow stronger that voice in the back of my head which tells me what to do. I will listen to my conscious and my subconscious and know how to read both in order to get the truth. I will always be prepared to have to face myself and look deep within my character to get to the root of my issues.

Narrator pauses for 3 seconds

Narrator: I will continue to do this because it is going to help me to lose weight. I will always look for ways to improve the natural methods that I can use to shed the pounds. I am confident in my own abilities to say "no" when it is needed. I won't act on impulse and I will always do my best to control my emotions. The better I can have a handle on my emotions, the easier it will be to know what I need to do to reach my goals and achieve my dreams.

Narrator pauses for 3 seconds

Narrator: I am focused on myself. I am doing this for myself. I am taking care of myself.

Narrator pauses for 3 seconds

Narrator: Each promise that I make to myself is one that brings me closer to my goals. I can feel the air coming in and out of my body. I am focused on relaxing, because reducing my stress will be important in achieving my goals. I am making a dedication to my body.

Narrator pauses for 3 seconds

Narrator: I am going to provide my body with all of the healthy food, water, air, and sun that it can get. I am like a gorgeous plant that needs the attention it deserves to have a vibrant and healthy blossom. I am devoted to myself. I love myself. I love my body. I am going to take care of my body. I am ready for the future. I am not afraid. I am accepting of the bad. I am excited for what is to come.

Narrator pauses for 3 seconds

Narrator: Take in several deeper breaths, just focusing on your body, your promises, and your goals. As you begin to bring yourself into the conscious, slowly open your eyes, press your palms together at your chest, and smile.

Chapter 9
Stop Emotional Eating Hypnosis

Emotional hunger and physical hunger are two very different things. Many individuals may claim that they're just trying to fill their empty stomach whenever they're taking a ton of food out of the fridge. However, they may just be trying to fill their empty heart or at least, to take their mind of something.

It's easy for many to not see the differences, especially when they're really depressed, stressed out, and troubled. If you're still stuck in a cycle of emotional hunger, frustration, and negativity, you're encouraged to take note of the things explained below.

Mindless Eating Usually Follows After Emotional Hunger

Mindless eating is characterized by a lack of awareness of what's going into your body or the amount of food you're stuffing yourself with. After several hours, you may have already consumed a whole bag of chips or a whole pint of ice cream without paying much attention and without fully enjoying the meal. You're emotional, not necessarily hungry.

Even after you've eaten a huge amount of food, you can still go at it because your mind's not registering what has been happening for the past few hours. When you're physically hungry, though, you're usually more mindful of what you're doing. You're just responding to the hunger, not the emotional instability.

Emotional Hunger is Sudden

Emotional hunger does not follow a specific schedule. It will hit you instantly, filling you with a sense of urgency that's simultaneously overwhelming and very tempting. Since emotions are also quite difficult to manage and predict, emotional hunger can surprise you in many instances. On the other hand, physical hunger is gradual.

Unless you haven't eaten in a very long time, you wouldn't want to eat as soon as possible. The hunger builds up because since your last meal this morning, you haven't had anything to eat. There's still an hour away before lunch break and your stomach's already rumbling a bit.

For example, you broke up with a long-time boyfriend or girlfriend. The immense sadness can lead you to consume a ton of potato chips and gallons of ice cream in the next few days.

You're not necessarily hungry, but your emotions have immediately kicked into gear, pushing you to eat despite the relative fullness. You may have seen a number of people who have put on a few pounds just a few days after their "personal tragedy." They quickly turned to food for comfort, hence the term "Comfort Food."

Being Full Won't Satisfy Emotional Hunger

Physical hunger can be satisfied when you've had your fill. After a healthy amount of food, you can continue being productive or doing various activities. On the other hand, emotional hunger continues to demand more and more. You're led to eat more because the bad or negative feelings haven't been addressed yet.

You're so focused on drowning your sorrows and disappointments with different types of "Comfort Food" that you forget about what your body actually needs. You're already full if you'll consider your physical needs, but your heart and mind aren't done yet. For so many reasons, they won't be done until you gain much weight; until you see what you've become because of emotional hunger.

Once you're full, but you're body's still searching for more food, consider the possibility of being emotionally hungry. Some people fall into a dangerous cycle of binge eating because they don't want to admit that they're emotionally troubled. They turn to food because they think they're just hungrier than usual. This isn't the case most of the time, though.

The fact that food can give you a good feeling makes it a formidable adversary in some cases, especially if you're prohibited to consume certain types of food due to health risks. There are other ways to satisfy your emotional needs and it's not through food.

Specific Comfort Foods are sought during Emotional Hunger

Physical hunger can be satisfied by virtually any type of food. Those who are simply hungry can get by with a vegetable salad with steamed tuna. Basically, healthy food are also considered—most likely even preferred more than unhealthy choices. You just want to respond to the hunger and get to such a goal in a healthy manner. Emotional hunger craves for specific and usually unhealthy snacks.

Your goal isn't to deal with the hunger, but to escape or cover up the pain you're feeling. For some, it's not necessarily pain, but a sense of helplessness or a couple of frustrations.

It's essentially the negativity that you're trying to defeat with positive feeling you're getting from the delicious cheese pizza or vanilla mint ice cream you're eating.

Guilt, Regret, or Shame Usually Follow After Emotional Hunger

People know what's bad and good for them. When they make healthy choices with regard to food, they are filled with satisfaction and genuine joy because they know they're taking good care of themselves. They eat only when they are hungry and they don't let their emotions dictate their food choices.

Sadly, for those who are emotionally hungry, guilt, regret, and shame can become frequent companions. After you finish that large bag of chips or that extra-large coke, you're filled with so much regret because you know it's not right. You're guilty because once again, you've allowed yourself to get caught up in the moment. You're also ashamed because you weren't strong enough to make the right decision.

There's one thing you have to know: everyone is prone to emotional hunger. Some are actually doing it unconsciously. No matter how old or young you are and what your circumstances may be, binge eating is a constant option.

Now that you have a better idea of what the differences are between physical or typical hunger and an emotional one, you can better explore the concept. You can now identify what is binge eating and what is not. The next step is to know the different causes of such an unhealthy activity.

The Causes of Emotional Eating

Childhood Habits

Look back at your experiences with food as a child. How did your parents associate food or eating to various circumstances in your life? If you were rewarded with food whenever you did something good or amazing, then you must have unconsciously considered food as a reward for good behavior.

Another way of looking at it is if your parents gave you sweets or a tasty meal whenever you were feeling down. In the early years, one's perspective regarding the role of food in his life is primarily influenced by his parents or guardians. Essentially, the overall view of the family towards food also creates a foundation for the young one's view of food when he grows older.

Emotionally-based childhood eating behaviors, which later on develop into habits, usually extend to adulthood. It's also actually possible for someone to eat based on nostalgic feelings. Eating because you remember how your dad grilled a couple of patties for you when you were younger definitely feels good.

At one point in your childhood, you may have baked a cake with your sweet mother. This may be why you're also eating a lot of pastries right now. You're very troubled and it's these types of food that help you feel secure. Many people want to feel like a child again, particularly during difficult moments.

Influence of Social Activities

One good way of relieving stress is to meet with your close friends or loved ones. Their presence and their tolerance of your food choices give a great feeling. You feel at home with them and because they may also be eating due to emotional hunger, you may end up doing the same.

There's a high tendency that overeating may occur because you're in the company of overeaters. You just decide to do what they're doing because all of you are going through tough challenges as well. You may want to empathize with them.

Another reason why overeating or binge eating may occur during social gatherings is nervousness. Things can get even worse if you're encouraged by your loved ones to eat a lot. They don't mind your current body mass because they love you too much to see you not eat and just sit at a corner.

When people go home to their families after being away for a very long time, the immense feeling of joy and relief can also cause them to consume a ton of food. They're not necessarily sad, but the occasion itself causes them to be so emotional, which can lead them to overeat.

Food turns into a medicine, which isn't really as effective as it's viewed to be. People just want to bury their negative emotions under huge pile of food. When they break up with someone, they turn to food. When they lose one of their loved ones, they think of the best possible way to stuff themselves up. When things don't go according to plan, a local binge eater shows his immense faith in the local supermarket and his great adoration for his refrigerator.

When you're stuffed with food, you feel like all the negativity just disappears, but they don't. When you stuff yourself to the point where you gain weight—when you apparently don't want to—you're just filled with a whole new batch of negative emotions.

As the binge eating continues, a very sturdy habit is formed.

This means the person will just get used to filling himself up when he has a problem. According to psychologists, a habit can be formed in just 21 days or 3 weeks. So if you've just started your binge eating journey, there's much time for positive transformation.

A Feeling of Emptiness or Extreme Boredom

Some people eat a ton of food just because they're bored. When they have nothing to do, they most likely don't even try to look for some activity to keep themselves busy. Boredom is sometimes a sign of laziness.

Basically, since an individual doesn't want to do what he's supposed to do, he ends up feeling empty. Instead of using this time to be productive or to help himself, he turns to food. This behavior can also turn into a habit if not detected, admitted, and addressed promptly.

If one delves into the matter more deeply, he'll see that boredom can also be considered as "free time," which can be utilized in a way that can help him and other people. Instead of opening the refrigerator whenever you have nothing to do or you're not in the mood yet to work on something, look for a better alternative. An empty space can be effectively filled by making the right or rational decisions, not emotional ones.

Have you ever noticed that stress can also make you hungry? It's actually not just in your head. Having chronic stress in this past-faced and chaotic world often leads to increased levels of cortisol, the stress hormone. Cortisol will trigger cravings for salty, sweet, and high-fat foods. These types of food will give you a burst of energy and pleasure, which is why they're so tempting to consume. The more stressed out you are, the more likely it is for you to turn to unhealthy food.

Unfortunately, so many things can act as stressors, so it's also a challenge for several people to handle themselves. At the workplace, school, and even at home, certain things stress people out. Avoiding stress would be another issue altogether, but making wise decisions on how to manage yourself during tense situations can make a difference.

You may not be able to control the circumstances you face at all times, but you can choose peace over turmoil and healthy living to unhealthy food choices. Know now that stress can turn most people into binge eaters. With this knowledge at hand, you can start being aware of yourself when you're in a pinch.

Using Awareness or Mindfulness to Beat Emotional Eating

You either eat with your emotions or with your mind. You can't really work with both. This is why mindful eating is considered to be the exact opposite of emotional eating. Awareness is a powerful tool in defeating binge eating. Once you become less emotional and more rational with regard to problem-solving or self-management, you'll be able to overcome this seemingly unbeatable foe.

You simply have to start with the identification of the triggers of emotional hunger. After that, you should look for better alternatives. As you work on these, you're also encouraged to savor the eating experience. Lastly, remember to live in the present.

Identify Triggers of Emotional Hunger

Many things can trigger emotional eating. Basically, whatever triggers your emotional outbursts or whatever fills you with negativity are the same factors that influence your diet. It may be a bit challenging to accomplish this step, but you can seek assistance from your loved ones.

You can do it, though. You just have to believe in your ability to not be biased when assessing yourself. Be more observant of your day-to-day activities and regard your problems through positive lenses.

Push pessimism away because this will hinder you from seeing the picture clearly. Instead of thinking that you'll just end up counting your problems, see it as an effective method of analyzing your enemies so that you can take them down. Great soldiers or warriors are aware of what they're feeling during various circumstances. They know what they should do because they look at each and every detail.

They're familiar with their weaknesses and it's this knowledge that enables them to turn such frailties into specialties or strengths. Whether it's stress, depression, a lack of validation or approval from your peers, or tension inside the household, the triggers of emotional hunger must be identified.

Find Alternatives to Address Negative Emotions

Emotional eating isn't the only path towards relief. Actually, it's not even a good path to begin with. Instead of eating to your heart's content whenever you're feeling down, look for other ways to lift yourself up. The greatest solutions to emotional hunger are of love.

This essentially means that if you do things that you're passionate about, you can feel more fulfilled and satisfied. The list of things that can make you happy certainly isn't only filled with different types of food. You will find other things to do in your free time and during those very difficult moments.

The alternatives need not be expensive. They don't even have to cost you a dime. Simply meditating a few times a week, talking to a good friend, or taking a walk at the park every day can take the blues away.

It's also advisable that you don't spend too much time in the kitchen whenever you're down. As you seek to be liberated from the clutches of emotional hunger, you must willingly distance yourself from temptation. The farther you are from your refrigerator, the better.

Savor the Eating Experience

Some say that obesity isn't a huge concern in France because they know how to enjoy their food. They're able to avoid a wider waistline by having a wider grin whenever they're eating. Generally, the French enjoy eating as much as they have fun cooking a variety of healthy and hearty meals.

You may not be a professional cook or chef, but you can choose to savor the eating experience whenever you're at home or when you're eating out. You can have fun eating, exploring the different flavors and textures of the meal before you.

Binge eaters "enjoy" food in a different way. They use it to conceal serious emotional struggles. Instead of eating to be healthy and to do away with their hunger, they use food to break out of their gloomy state. Unfortunately, they're not really free. If you seek freedom, one effective way of achieving it is to savor every bite and to not rush to the refrigerator during a crisis. Enjoy your salad, steak, or whatever it is in front of you. Don't eat more than you're supposed to because your sadness and disappointments won't vacate your heart just because your stomach's filled with so much food.

Chapter 10
Weight Loss Hypnosis

This hypnosis is going to be a way that will validate your weight loss goals. You will be able to recognize how relaxing and being peaceful throughout the weight loss process makes it easier to keep the pounds off. Keep an open mind with this, and remember to let thoughts flow naturally into your brain as if they were your own.

Hypnosis for Natural Weight Loss

You know how to relax your body. You are an expert at making sure that your limbs can hang freely without tension. We need to let our minds relax now.

Don't just let your body feel like jelly floating through water. Let your mind be as malleable in this process too. With hypnosis, you have to let others into your head for just a moment. So allow your thoughts to flow freely and don't put any pressure on yourself to think a certain thing. Focus now on your breath.

Breathe in for five and out for five. Breathe in through your nose and out through your mouth. This is a way that's going to help make sure that you are focused on healthy living. Breathe in for one, two, three, four, and five, and out for five, four, three, two, and one.

Now we're going to do something a little different. Breathe in for five and then out for one long second. This time, we're only going to breathe in and out through your nose. Breathe in through your nose for one, two, three, four, and five, and out for one and a long and forceful breath.

You are slowly breathing in new air, and then you forcefully push it out as fast as you can. Breathe in for one, two, three, four, and five, and out for one with a quick snap. This way, you focus your breathing and make it easier for the air to flow in and out of your body.

You are going to want to snap your attention on nothing. You can look ahead of you now, but make sure that you get all of your sights out. On the count of three, you're going to snap your eyes closed and also breathe out at the same time.

So look around you and breathe in for one, two, three, four, and five. Now quickly shut your eyes and breathe out in one long breath.

You can go back to regular breathing now but continue to focus on breathing in through your nose and out through your mouth. Try to do it in a pattern of five, but don't get too hung up on the strict structure. Instead, you'll want to focus on letting your thoughts come into your brain as if they were your own.

Keep your mind focused and breathe in. In front of you, in your mind, only with your eyes closed, see the emergence of a spinning wheel. This wheel has nothing special about it. It is simply silver with rubber tires, and it is spinning fast. It is not attached to anything. It is simply a spinning wheel. It spins faster and faster and faster. Stare directly at the silver center. Notice how it continues to cycle through quickly.

Now that tire is turning into a circle of water. The water is flowing around as if it were a washing machine with water being spun in a circle.

The water is spinning and spinning. It is splashing against itself, but it is all still contained within this one simple silver circle. Continue to look at the center. There is nothing else around; everything is black. Notice this silver spinning water. It goes over and over and over in a simple cycle in a simple loop. Focus on the center again as we count for your breathing. Breathe in for one, two, three, four, and five, and out for five, four, three, two, and one.

Suddenly, on the count of three, this spinning cycle is going to snap into every corner of your mind. You are going to be engulfed in this spinning water.

One, two, and three.

You are now in the water. You see around you that you are on a calm beach. The water is not spinning anymore and is completely serene and clear. You walk towards the edge of the beach. You see it now that the water is slapping against the shore. This is the way that it was spinning around in circles in your mind.

No longer is it spinning now, and it is simply a normal ocean slapping against the beach. You can feel the water dripping off your skin, but the sun above you is already drying out. The sun is a vibrant yellow, and it casts a warm glow over your body. The sun kisses you at the top of your head and spreads down all the way to the tip of your toes. You look down at your feet and see that they're submerged in the sand. There is still water gently coming over and washing against your feet. You move your toes upwards, and they break through some of the sand, only for it to quickly form over them again. As the water smooths it out, you look ahead of you and breathe in again. You breathe in for one, two, three, four, and five, and out for five, four, three, two, and one, and notice all of these smells that come in with that. You breathe again for one, two, three, four, and five, and out for five, four, three, two, and one. You feel refreshed, energized, and free.

You are natural, pure, clean, and clear. You are part of this beach now with your feet stuck in the sand. You are like a tree with roots deep under the surface.

You decide now to sit down. You let your bum sink into the sand a little bit more as well. Water continues to emerge around you now like a warm blanket, all the way up to your hips. It keeps you feeling completely centered and pure on the now.

You look around you, to your right and left, and see that there are plenty of rocks. These, of course, don't hurt you. They just simply are part of the sand. You dig your fingers into the sand, a little bit feeling the cold packed down underneath the initial warm on the top of the surface. You dig out a rock and see that it is flat and smooth. You clear a little bit of this rock off using water as it passes over. You throw the rock quickly and sharply against the top of the water and watch as it jumps. It was a nice skipping rock that effortlessly glided across the top.

You do this a few more times with other smooth and flat rocks that surround you. It is a reminder of how you can manipulate nature.

The water is getting higher and higher now, and you are chest-deep in the water. It is perfectly warm and calm, bringing plenty of waves back to the surface. You want to feel the sun on your skin again now, so you decide to stand up.

You walk across the sand, now in the dry area. Sand begins to stick to your legs, but still, it is nice and warm. You walk across, feeling your feet sink deep in. Each new step you take, the bottom of your foot is hot from the surface of the sand. It adjusts quickly as it sinks down, and you feel a sensation over and over again as you continue to walk. You see ahead of you that there is what looks to be a sandcastle. As you get closer and closer, you see that there is no castle at all. It is simply a wall that somebody has built with the sand. You decide to walk all the way through this wall now.

No longer is there something that is going to block off part of the beach. It was simply made by sand, so it was easy for you to destroy with your feet and legs only. You recognize that this is a representation of the walls that you have built around yourself. No longer are you going to let yourself be afraid of the things that you want. You can't just be comfortable with the situation you're in anymore. Being comfortable does not always mean being happy. You want to be able to feel completely fresh and pure. You're not attached to the things that you used to be or the person that used to keep your mind stuck in the same situations over and over again.

You sit in the middle of the now-destroyed wall and look out on the beach again. The sun continues to send warm feelings all across your skin.

You breathe in deeply, feeling this ocean air fill your body once again. These oceans are responsible for so much. They are the life force that keeps everybody moving. We take fish from the ocean, and it helps us travel and carry things across waters. You breathe. All of this is a reminder of the incredible world that you're a part of.

While your problems and issues are valid, this is also a reminder of how small some things that seem like such big deals to us really are in the grand scheme of things. There is a great and powerful force that exists just within the world alone.

You are an important part of this, and it is a reminder of the incredible and powerful person that you are.

The sun is setting, so you decide to go for one last and final dip before you don't have the chance anymore. You don't want to swim in the dark, so you decide to wade in a little bit and get your last dose of ocean water right now. You walk in, and the water is all the way up to your hip. You can look down and see the ocean floor because the water is so clear.

You don't really see any fish, but you can see the old shells left over by different crabs or other ocean critters.

You walk a little bit further, and now the water is up to your chest. The waves are so gentle you barely feel them. It's almost as if you were in a deep and warm bath because the water is so relaxing.

You decide to lift your legs up now. Floating on top of the water, you simply move around, letting the waves take you where you need to go. If you go out too far from the shore or off to the side too much, you can gently guide yourself back to where you want to be with a simple arm or leg movement.

You are simply free in the water, almost as if you're flying through the sky. There is no gravity in this moment. You breathe in and out, in and out. The water is surrounding you now. A few droplets will get on your face here and there as the water continues to splash around you, but nothing too extreme.

You close your eyes for just a moment, letting water wash over your face. You are clean, pure, natural, and energized in this moment. Breathe in for five and out for five. Breathe in for five and out for five. Everything around you is turning black. Darkness begins to consume you once again, and you realize you are now back in your bed on the couch, ready to start a new life.

You are pure, energized, and prepared. As we count on from 20, you will be out of this hypnosis. You can then either drift asleep or move on to another mental exercise.

Chapter 11
Eat Healthy With Subliminal Hypnosis

Make yourself comfortable.

Find the perfect sleep position.

Inhale through your nose and exhale through your mouth.

Again inhale through your nose and this time as you exhale close your eyes.

Repeat this one more time and relax.

Sharpen your breathing focus.

Find stillness in every breath you take, relieve yourself from any tension and relax.

Let your body relax, soften your heart, quiet your anxious mind and open to whatever you experience without fighting.

Simply allow your thoughts and experiences to come and go without grasping at them.

Reduce any stress, anxiety, or negative emotions you might have, cool down become deeply and comfortably relaxed.

That's fine.

And as you continue to relax then you can begin the process of reprogramming your mind for your weight loss success because with the right mindset, then you can think positively about what you want to achieve. It begins with changing your mindset and attitude, because the key to losing weight all starts in the mind. One of the very first things you must throw out the window (figuratively) before you start your journey to weight loss is negativity. Negative thinking will just lead you nowhere. It will only pull your moods down which might trigger emotional eating. Thus, you'll eat more, adding up to that unwanted weight instead of losing it. Remember that you must need to break your old bad habits and one of them is negative self-talk. You need to change your negative mental views and turn them into positive ones. For example, instead of telling yourself after a few days of workout that nothing is happening or changing, tell yourself that you have done a set of physical activities you have never imagine you can or will do. Make it a point to pat yourself on the back for every little progress you make every day, may it be five additional crunches from what you did yesterday. Understand and accept that this process is a complete transformation, a metamorphosis if you will. This understanding is going to make the process smoother, and less painful.

Aside from being positive, you should also be realistic. Don't expect an immediate change in your body. Keep in mind that losing weight is not an overnight thing. It is a long term process and gradual progress. Set and focus on your goals to keep that negativity at bay. Losing weight needs consistent reminders and focus on proper mental preparations. Always keep yourself motivated. Train yourself to think positive all the time.

Don't compare yourself to others, because it will not help you attain your goals in losing weight. First and foremost, keep in mind that each one of us has different body types and compositions. There is a certain diet that may work on you, but not so much for the others. Possibly, some people might need more carbohydrates in their diet, while you might need to drop that and add more protein in your meals. Each one of us is unique. Therefore, your diet plan will surely differ from the person next to you.

Comparing yourself to other people's progress is just a negative thought and will just be unhelpful to you. Remember, always keep a positive outlook and commit to it before you start your diet. For the sake of your long-term success, leave the comparison trap. You're not exactly like the people you idolize and they're not exactly like you and that's perfectly fine. Accept that, embrace that and move on with your personal goals.

Be realistic in setting your goals. Think about small and easy to achieve goals that will guide you towards a long term of healthy lifestyle changes. Your goals should be healthy for your body. If you want to truly lose weight and keep it off, it will be a slow uphill battle, with occasional dips and times you'll want to quit. If you expect progress too fast, you will eventually not be able to reach your goals and become discouraged. Don't add extra obstacles for yourself, plan your goals carefully.

If possible, try to find someone who has similar goals as you and work on them together. Two is always better than one, and having someone who understands what you are undergoing can be such a relief! An added benefit of having a partner-in-crime (or several) is that you can always hold each other accountable. Accountability is one thing that is easy to start being lax after the first few weeks of a new weight loss program, especially if results aren't quite where you want them to be.

Write down a realistic timetable that you can follow. Start a journal about your daily exercises and meal plan. You can cross out things that you have done already or add new ones along the way. Plot your physical activities. Make time and mark your calendar with daily physical activities. Try to incorporate at least a 15-minute workout on your busy days.

When you become aware of a thought or belief that pins the blame for your extra weight on something outside yourself, if you can find examples of people who've overcome that same cause, realize that it's decision time for you. Choose for yourself whether this is a thought you want to embrace and accept. Does this thought support you living your best life? Does it move you toward your goals, or does it give you an excuse not to go after them?

If you determine your thought no longer serves you, you get to choose another thought instead. Instead of pointing to some external, all-powerful cause for you being overweight, you can choose something different. Track your progress by writing down your step count or workouts daily to keep track of your progress.

Celebrate and embrace your results. Since the path to a healthy lifestyle is mostly hard work and discipline, try to reward yourself for every progress even if it is small. Treat yourself for a day of pampering, travel to a place you have been wanting to visit, go hiking, have a movie date with friends or get a new pair of shoes. These kinds of rewards provide you gratification and accomplishments that will make you keep going. Little things do count and little things also deserve recognition. But keep in mind that your rewards should not compromise your diet plan.

You can also do something like joining an athletic event, a fun run, where you can meet new people that share the same ideals of a healthy lifestyle. You get to learn more about weight loss from others and also share your knowledge. You need to find a source of motivation and keep that source of motivation fresh in your mind so you don't forget why you embarked on this journey to begin with.

As you focus on your journey of weight loss, keep your stress at bay because too much stress is harmful for the body in many ways, but it also can cause people to gain weight. When the body is under stress, the body will automatically release many hormones and among one of them is cortisol. When the body is under duress and stress, cortisol is released, is can ignite the metabolism, for a period of time. However, if the body remains in stressful conditions, the hormone cortisol will continue to be released, and actually slow down the metabolism resulting in weight gain.

Everyone experiences stress; there is just no getting around that fact. However, minimizing stressors, as well as learning how to manage the stress in your life will not only help you with you with losing weight, but it will also make a more attractive you! High stress in anyone's life often brings out the worst in people. When you are trying to get a man, you want them to see the best of you, not the stressed out you. While you are decreasing your stress level, you will want to increase the amount of sleep you get each night. Lack of sleep is a link to weight gain and because of this, ensuring adequate and appropriate sleep is crucial when trying to lose weight. Sleep is vital for the well being of the body, and the ability for the mind to function, but it is also related to maintaining weight. If you are tired, make sure you sleep, rest or relax, so you are not prone to gaining weight. When a person gets more sleep, the hormone leptin will rise and when this happens the appetite decreases which will also decrease body weight.

Gratitude is important in this journey because it teaches you how to make peace with your body, no matter what shape, size or weight it has at the moment. It makes you look at your body with full acceptance and love, saying: "I'm grateful for my body the way it is." It stops you from beating yourself up for being overweight, unhealthy or out of shape. Be grateful for this learning experience, accept yourself the way you are, and take massive action to get your balance back.

When you express gratitude, you vibrate on a higher energy level, you are positive and happy, and you are simply in the state of satisfaction.

The more things you can find to be grateful for during your weight loss journey, the easier it will be to maintain a positive attitude and keep your motivation up.

It will also get you past those tough moments when you are feeling demotivated to take action and stick to the exercising or eating plan.

This means that you start expressing gratitude for the aspects of your body you would like to have, as if you already have them now. Be grateful for your sexy legs and slim waist. Be grateful for your increased energy levels and strength. Be grateful for the ability to wear smaller clothes. You get the drill. Feel the positive energy of gratitude flowing through your body as you imagine these things are true. By going through this exercise you'll notice the positive change in your thought patterns.

With the level of personal growth, you will achieve and the habits you will change on this session of hypnosis, you will feel like a completely different person. You will have more power, self–confidence and love yourself more than you ever thought possible before. That's change from the inside out. That's what lasts. And, at the end of the day, that's what truly matters.

Take a deep breath and allow your breath to return its natural rate as you return to your normal consciousness.

As you continue to breath, note that, right now, in this moment, you have no worries. You are just a relaxed body. Any distractions that arise while you tell yourself this can wait.

Repeat the following phrases:

I am relaxed

I am balanced

I can deal with any worries later

I am relaxed

I am balanced

The whole earth supports you in your relaxation and balance. Feel yourself supported and held.

Feel that everything you have done in your life has brought you to this moment without errors or mistakes.

This moment is perfect.

When you feel doubt, say hello to it and let it know it can't distract you from your purpose.

You are relaxed

You are balanced

You can deal with all doubts and worries.

Know that you can achieve this at any time because you are supported and held in balance.

Thank yourself for taking this time to connect with your body and balance.

Open your eyes and gently move your hands and feet.

Three eyes open and completely awake.

Chapter 12
Loss Weight Fast And Naturally With Hypnosis

Hypnosis As A Means Of Losing Weight

Hypnosis might be best known as the gathering stunt used to make people move the chicken in front of an audience. However, an ever-increasing number of people go to the psychological control system to help them make more beneficial choices and get in shape. A valid example: The consuming fewer calories master changed to spellbinding when Georgia, 28, chose she required to shed the 30 pounds she put on after foot medical procedure in 2009. The technique for mind-control had helped her in the past to conquer a dread of flying, and she trusted that it would likewise enable her to make good dieting practices.

Georgia subsequently decided to engage in hypnotherapy to help her lose weight. In short, each session was focused on planting positive thoughts in her mind such as knowing when to stop eating and finding the best way to help her stop overeating based on emotional reactions. The treatment proved to be progressively effective as she was able to curb her appetite and manage her eating habits more effectively. She was able to drop the weight that she wanted based on improving her overall eating habits, curbing her cravings and limiting the instances of binge eating.

Mesmerizing is for anybody searching for a mellow way to get thinner and make smart dieting a propensity. Is it safe to say that it isn't for one person? Any individual who needs a quick fix. It expects time to reframe issue thoughts regarding sustenance Georgia reveals to her trance inducer eight times each year, and it took a month before she started to see a genuine change. "The weight fell gradually and definitely, without tremendous adjustments in my way of life. I was all the while eating out many times each week, yet regularly sending plates back with sustenance on them! I truly tasted my sustenance unexpectedly, investing energy in flavors and surfaces. It was as though I had begun my illicit affection relationship with nourishment, no one, but I could get thinner," she said.

Spellbinding isn't planned to be a "diet," but instead an apparatus to help you prevail with regards to eating and practicing nutritious sustenance, states Traci Stein, Ph.D., MPH, an ASCH-ensured clinical entrancing wellbeing clinician and previous Director of Integrative Medicine at Columbia University's Department of Surgery. "Spellbinding enables people to encounter what they feel when they are ground-breaking, fit, and indirection in a multi-tactile way and conquer their psychological hindrances to accomplish those goals," she guarantees. "In particular, trance can help people unravel the hidden mental issues that reason them to abhor work out, experience extreme longings, gorge during the evening, or eat heedlessly. It empowers them to recognize the triggers and incapacitate them.

"As a general rule, it is valuable not to consider mesmerizing an eating regimen by any stretch of the imagination, says Joshua E. Syna, MA, LCDC, an authorized trance specialist at the Houston Hypnosis Center." It works since it changes their perspective about sustenance and eating and empowers them to figure out how to be increasingly quiet and agreeable in their life. So as opposed to being a passionate answer for sustenance and eating, it turns into a reasonable answer for craving, and new personal conduct standards are being made that enable the person to adapt to sentiments and life, "he depicts." Hypnosis works for weight reduction since it enables the person to isolate nourishment and eat from their enthusiastic lives.

Dr. Stein proposes that utilizing at-home independently directed sound projects produced by a gifted subliminal specialist (search for an ASCH affirmation) is alright for people with no other emotional wellness issues. Be that as it may, be careful with all the new online market applications, one investigation found that most applications are untested and regularly make affected cases about their viability that can't be substantiated.

What Hypnosis Feels Like

Forget what you found in movies and front of an audience is more like a treatment session than a carnival stunt. "Trance is a community-oriented encounter and at all times ought to be very much educated and agreeable," says Dr. Stein.

What's more, she adds to individuals stressed over being fooled into accomplishing something odd or hurtful, even under entrancing on the off chance that you would prefer truly not to accomplish something, you won't. "Consideration is simply focused," she portrays. "Normally everybody goes into light daze articulations a few times each day-accept about when you daydream while a companion shares everything about their vacation and trance just figures out how to think that internal consideration in a supportive way." Dispelling the legend that entrancing feels weird or terrifying from the patient's side, Georgia claims she generally felt exceptionally clear and leveled out.

There were even entertaining occasions such as envisioning steps on the scale and seeing the heaviness of her target. "My excessively inventive personality needed to envision initially taking off all garments, all of the gems, my watch, and barrette before hopping on naked. Any other individual does that, or is it just me?" (No, it's not simply you, Georgia!)

It's not intrusive, it functions admirably with other weight reduction medications, and it doesn't include any pills, powders, or different enhancements. Nothing occurs even from a pessimistic standpoint, placing it in the camp "may help, can't hurt." But Dr. Stein concedes that one drawback is there: cost. Expenses every hour contrast dependent on your place, yet for helpful spellbinding systems, it differs from $100-$250 an hour and when you see the specialist for a month or two once per week or more that can include rapidly. What's more, trance isn't secured by most insurance agencies. Be that as it may, Dr. Stein proposes it very well may be secured whenever utilized as a major aspect of a greater arrangement for psychological wellness treatment, so check with your provider.

A surprising perk of weight loss hypnosis isn't only a psychological thing, it's likewise a medicinal component, says Peter LePort, MD, a bariatric specialist, and Memorial Care Center for Obesity's therapeutic chief in California. "You should initially adapt to any hidden metabolic or natural weight increase causes yet utilizing spellbinding can kick start sound propensities while that is no joke," he proposes. Furthermore, there is another great advantage of utilizing spellbinding: "The component of reflection can diminish pressure and lift mindfulness, which can likewise help with weight reduction," he added.

How Hypnosis Aids In Weight Loss

There is an amazing measure of logical research that takes a gander at the viability of weight reduction mesmerizing, and a lot of it is sure. One of the underlying 1986 research found that overweight females utilizing a mesmerizing project shed 17 pounds contrasted with 0.5 pounds for females just advised to watch what they ate. A mesmerizing weight reduction study meta-investigation during the 1990s found that members who utilized trance lost more than twice as much weight as the individuals who didn't. Also, an examination in 2014 found that females who utilized entrancing were improving their weight, BMI, eating conduct, and even certain parts of self-perception.

In any case, it's not all uplifting news: A Stanford study in 2012 found that about a fourth of individuals just can't be mesmerized, and it has nothing to do with their characters, as opposed to basic conviction. Or maybe, the minds of certain individuals simply don't appear to work that way. "In case you're not inclined to staring off into space, you regularly think that it's difficult to stall out in a book or endure a motion picture, and don't believe you're innovative, you may be one of the individuals for whom trance isn't functioning admirably," says Dr. Stein.

Georgia is one of the examples of overcoming adversity. She guarantees it helped her lose the extra pounds as well as helped her keep them off also. After six years, she kept her weight reduction joyfully, now and then returning in with her trance specialist when she requires a boost.

Understanding The Hypnotic Gastric Band And How It Works

Gastric band hypnotherapy is a technique used to propose that you have a gastric band connected around your stomach to the intuitive to enable you to get more fit.

Gastric band medical procedure, thought about a final retreat, incorporates fitting a band around the upper segment of the stomach. This confines the amount of sustenance that you can expend physically, advancing weight reduction. It is an activity and, in this manner, involves future dangers and confusion.

Hypnotherapy of the gastric band or fitting a' virtual gastric band' doesn't include the medical procedure. Trance inducers utilize this technique to get the subliminal to think a gastric band has been fitted. The objective is to believe that you have had the physical activity on an oblivious level and that your stomach has diminished in size.

There is no medical procedure or medicine associated with the procedure, and it is thoroughly secure. In this segment, we will explore what is engaged with gastric band hypnotherapy, how it works, and on the off chance that it can work for you or not.

What Is A Gastric Band?

A stomach band is a silicone flexible apparatus utilized in weight reduction medical procedure. To create a modest pack over the gadget, the band is put around the upper part of the belly. This restrains the amount of sustenance that can be put away in the stomach area, making eating enormous amounts hard.

A gastric band will likely constrain the amount of sustenance that an individual can expend physically, making them feel full in the wake of eating next to no to advance weight reduction. It is a final hotel for most people who have this medical procedure after endeavoring for other weight reduction systems. Like any medical procedure, there are perils in fitting a gastric band.

Chapter 13
100 Positive Affirmations For Weight Loss

According to dietitians, the success of dieting is greatly influenced by how people talk about lifestyle changes for others and for themselves.

The use of "I should" or "I must" is to be avoided whenever possible. Anyone who says, "I shouldn't eat French fries" or "I have to get a bite of chocolate" will feel that they have no control over the events. Instead, if you say "I prefer" to leave the food, you will feel more power and less guilt. The term "dieting" should be avoided. Good nutrition should be seen as a permanent lifestyle change. For example, the correct wording is, "I've changed my eating habits" or "I'm eating healthier".

Diets are fattening. Why?

The body needs fat. Our body wants to live, so it stores fat. Removing this amount of fat from the body is not an easy task as the body protects against weight loss. During starvation, our bodies switch to a 'saving flame', burning fewer calories to avoid starving. Those who are starting to lose weight are usually optimistic, as, during the first week, they may experience 1-3 kg (2-7 lbs.) of weight loss, which validates their efforts and suffering. Their body, however, has deceived them very well because it actually does not want to break down fat. Instead, it begins to break down muscle tissue. At the beginning of dieting, our bodies burn sugar and protein, not fat. Burned sugar removes a lot of water out of the body; that's why we experience amazing results on the scale. It should take about seven days for our body to switch to fat burning. Then our body's alarm bell rings. Most diets have a sad end: reducing your metabolic rate to a lower level. This means that if you only eat a little more afterward, you regain all the weight you have lost previously. After dieting, the body will make special efforts to store fat for the next impending famine. What to do to prevent such a situation?

We must understand what our soul needs. Those who really desire to have success must first and foremost change their spiritual foundation. It is important to pamper our souls during a period of weight loss. All overweight people tend to rag on themselves for eating forbidden food, "I ate too much again. My willpower is so weak!" If you have ever tried to lose weight, you know these thoughts very well.

Imagine a person very close to you who has gone through a difficult time while making mistakes from time to time. Are we going to scold or try to help and motivate them? If we really love them, we would instead comfort them and try to convince them to continue. No one tells their best friend that they are weak, ugly, or bad, just because they are struggling with their weight. If you wouldn't say it to your friend, don't do so to yourself either! Let us be aware of this: during weight loss, our soul needs peace and support. All bad opinions, even if they are only expressed in thought, are detrimental and divert us from our purpose. You must support yourself with positive reinforcement. There is no place for the all or nothing principle. A single piece of cake will not ruin your entire diet. Realistic thinking is more useful than disaster theory. A cookie is not the end of the world. Eating should not be a reward. Cakes should not make up for a bad day. If you are generally a healthy consumer, eat some goodies sometimes because of its delicious taste and to pamper your soul.

I'll give you a list of a hundred positive affirmations you can use to reinforce your weight loss. I'll divide them into main categories based on the most typical situations for which you would need confirmation. You can repeat all of them whenever you need to, but you can also choose the ones that are more suitable for your circumstances. If you prefer to listen to them during meditation, you can record them with a piece of nice relaxing music in the background.

General affirmations to reinforce your wellbeing:

1. I'm grateful that I woke up today. Thank you for making me happy today.

2. Today is a very good day. I meet nice and helpful people, whom I treat kindly.

3. Every new day is for me. I live to make myself feel good. Today I just pick good thoughts for myself.

4. Something wonderful is happening to me today.

5. I feel good.

6. I am calm, energetic and cheerful.

7. My organs are healthy.

8. I am satisfied and balanced.

9. I live in peace and understanding with everyone.

10. I listen to others with patience.

11. In every situation, I find the good.

12. I accept and respect myself and my fellow human beings.

13. I trust myself, I trust my inner wisdom.

Do you often scold yourself? Then repeat the following affirmations frequently:

14. I forgive myself.

15. I'm good to myself.

16. I motivate myself over and over again.

17. I'm doing my job well.

18. I care about myself.

19. I am doing my best.

20. I am proud of myself for my achievements.

21. I am aware that sometimes I have to pamper my soul.

22. I remember that I did a great job this week.

23. I deserved this small piece of candy.

24. I let go of the feeling of guilt.

25. I release the blame.

26. Everyone is imperfect. I accept that I am too.

If you feel pain when you choose to avoid delicious food, then you need to motivate yourself with affirmations such as:

27. I am motivated and persistent.

28. I control my life and my weight.

29. I'm ready to change my life.

30. Changes make me feel better.

31. I follow my diet with joy and cheerfulness.

32. I am aware of my amazing capacities.

33. I am grateful for my opportunities.

34. Today I'm excited to start a new diet.

35. I always keep in mind my goals.

36. I imagine myself slim and beautiful.

37. Today I am happy to have the opportunity to do what I have long been postponing.

38. I possess the energy and will to go through my diet.

39. I prefer to lose weight instead of wasting time on momentary pleasures.

Here you can find affirmations that help you to change harmful convictions and blockages:

40. I see my progress every day.

41. I listen to my body's messages.

42. I'm taking care of my health.

43. I eat healthy food.

44. I love who I am.

45. I love how life supports me.

46. A good parking space, coffee, conversation. It's all for me today.

47. It feels good to be awake because I can live in peace, health, love.

48. I'm grateful that I woke up. I take a deep breath of peace and tranquility.

49. I love my body. I love being served by me.

50. I eat by tasting every flavor of the food.

51. I am aware of the benefits of healthy food.

52. I enjoy eating healthy food and being fitter every day.

53. I feel energetic because I eat well.

Many people are struggling with being overweight because they don't move enough. The very root of this issue can be a refusal to do exercises due to negative biases in our minds.

We can overcome these beliefs by repeating the following affirmations:

54. I like moving because it helps my body burn fat.

55. Each time I exercise, I am getting closer to having a beautiful, tight shapely body.

56. It's a very uplifting feeling of being able to climb up to 100 steps without stopping.

57. It's easier to have an excellent quality of life if I move.

58. I like the feeling of returning to my home tired but happy after a long winter walk.

59. Physical exercises help me have a longer life.

60. I am proud to have better fitness and agility.

61. I feel happier thanks to the happiness hormone produced by exercise.

62. I feel full thanks to the enzymes that produce a sense of fullness during physical exercises.

63. I am aware even after exercise, my muscles continue to burn fat, and so I lose weight while resting.

64. I feel more energetic after exercises.

65. My goal is to lose weight, therefore I exercise.

66. I am motivated to exercise every day.

67. I lose weight while I exercise.

Now, I am going to give you a list of generic affirmations that you can build in your own program:

68. I'm glad I'm who I am.

69. Today, I read articles and watch movies that make me feel positive about my diet progress.

70. I love when I'm happy.

71. I take a deep breath and exhale my fears.

72. Today I do not want to prove my truth, but I want to be happy.

73. I am strong and healthy. I'm fine and I'm getting better.

74. I am happy today because whatever I do, I find joy in it.

75. I pay attention to what I can become.

76. I love myself and am helpful to others.

77. I accept what I cannot change.

78. I am happy that I can eat healthy food.

79. I am happy that I have been changing my life with my new healthy lifestyle.

80. Today I do not compare myself to others.

81. I accept and support who I am and turn to myself with love.

82. Today I can do anything for my improvement.

83. I'm fine. I'm happy for life. I love who I am. I'm strong and confident.

84. I am calm and satisfied.

85. Today is perfect for me to exercise and being healthy.

86. I have decided to lose weight and I am strong enough to follow my will.

87. I love myself, so I want to lose weight.

88. I am proud of myself because I follow my diet program.

89. I see how much stronger I am.

90. I know that I can do it.

91. It is not my past but my present that defines me.

92. I am grateful for my life.

93. I am grateful for my body because it collaborates well with me.

94. Eating healthy foods supports me to get the best nutrients I need, to be in the best shape.

95. I eat only healthy foods, and I avoid processed foods.

96. I can achieve my weight loss goals.

97. All cells in my body are fit and healthy, and so am I.

98. I enjoy staying healthy and sustaining my ideal weight.

99. I feel that my body is losing weight right now.

100. I care about my body by exercising every day.

Chapter 14
Daily Habits For Weight Loss

Understanding Mindful Eating

There are various scopes of cautious eating techniques, some of them established in Zen and different kinds of Buddhism, others connected to yoga.

Here, we are taking a simple technique, and that is the primary concern.

My careful eating procedure is figuring out how to be cautious. Rather than eating carelessly, putting nourishment unknowingly in your mouth, not so much tasting the sustenance you eat, you see your thoughts, and feelings.

- Learn to be cautious: why you want to eat, and what emotions or requirements can trigger eating.

- What you eat, and whether it's solid.

- Look, smell, taste, feel the nourishment that you eat.

- How do you feel like when you taste it, how would you digest it, and go about your day?

- How complete you are previously, during, and in the wake of eating.

- During and in the wake of eating, your sentiments.

- Where the nourishment originated from, who could have developed it, the amount it could have suffered before it was killed, regardless of whether it was naturally developed, the amount it was handled, the amount it was broiled or overcooked, and so on.

This is an ability that you don't simply increase medium-term, a type of reflection. It takes practice, and there will be times when you neglect to eat mindfully, beginning, and halting. However, you can get generally excellent at this with exercise and consideration.

Mindful Eating Benefits

The upsides of eating mindfully are unimaginable and realizing these points of interest is fundamental as you think about the activity.

- When you're anxious, you figure out how to eat and stop when you're plunking down.

- You figure out how to taste nourishment and acknowledge great sustenance tastes.

- You start to see gradually that unfortunate nourishment isn't as scrumptious as you accepted, nor does it make you feel extremely pleasant.

- Because of the over three points, if you are overweight, you will regularly get more fit.

- You start arranging your nourishment and eating through the passionate issues you have. It requires somewhat more, yet it's basic.

- Social overeating can turn out to be less of an issue—you can eat mindfully while mingling, rehearsing, and not over-alimenting.

- You begin to appreciate the experience of eating more, and as an outcome, you will acknowledge life more when you are progressively present.

- It can transform into a custom of mindfulness that you anticipate.

- You learn for the day how nourishment impacts your disposition and vitality.

- You realize what fuel your training best with nourishment, and you work and play.

A Guide To Mindful Eating

Keeping up a contemporary, quick-paced way of life can leave a brief period to oblige your necessities. You are moving always starting with one thing then onto the next, not focusing on what your psyche or body truly needs. Rehearsing mindfulness can help you to comprehend those necessities.

When eating mindfulness is connected, it can help you recognize your examples and practices while simultaneously standing out to appetite and completion related to body signs.

Originating from the act of pressure decrease dependent on mindfulness, rehearsing mindfulness while eating can help you focus on the present minute instead of proceeding with ongoing and unacceptable propensities.

Careful eating is an approach to begin an internal looking course to help you become increasingly aware of your nourishment association and utilize that information to eat with joy.

The body conveys a great deal of information and information, so you can start settling on cognizant choices as opposed to falling into programmed — and regularly feeling driven — practices when you apply attention to the eating knowledge. You are better prepared to change your conduct once you become aware of these propensities.

Individuals that need to be cautious about sustenance and nourishment are asked to:

- Explore their inward knowledge about sustenance— different preferences

- Choose sustenance that please and support their bodies

- Accept explicit sustenance inclinations without judgment or self-analysis

- Practice familiarity with the indications of their bodies beginning to eat and quit eating.

General Principles Of Mindful Eating

One methodology to careful eating depends on the core values given by Rebecca J. Frey, Ph.D., and Laura Jean Cataldo, RN: tune in to the internal craving and satiety signs of your body Identify private triggers for careless eating, for example, social weights, amazing sentiments, and explicit nourishments.

Here are a couple of tips for getting you started.

- Start with one meal. It requires some investment to begin with any new propensity. It very well may be difficult to make cautious eating rehearses constantly. However, you can practice with one dinner or even a segment of a supper. Attempt to focus on appetite sign and sustenance choices before you start eating or sinking into the feelings of satiety toward the part of the arrangement—these are phenomenal approaches to begin a routine with regards to consideration.

- Remove view distractions place or turn off your phone in another space. Mood killers such the TV and PC and set away whatever else —, for example, books, magazines, and papers—that can divert you from eating. Give the feast before your complete consideration.

- Tune in your perspective when you start this activity, become aware of your attitude. Perceive that there is no right or off base method for eating, yet simply unmistakable degrees of eating background awareness. Focus your consideration on eating sensations. When you understand that your brain has meandered, take it delicately back to the eating knowledge.

- Draw in your senses with this activity. There are numerous approaches to explore. Attempt to investigate one nourishment thing utilizing every one of your faculties. When you put sustenance in your mouth, see the scents, surfaces, hues, and flavors. Attempt to see how the sustenance changes as you cautiously bite each nibble.

- Take as much time as necessary. Eating cautiously includes backing off, enabling your stomach related hormones to tell your mind that you are finished before eating excessively. It's a fabulous method to hinder your fork between chomps. Additionally, you will be better arranged to value your supper experience, especially in case you're with friends and family.

Rehearsing mindfulness in a bustling globe can be trying now and again; however, by knowing and applying these essential core values and techniques, you can discover approaches to settle your body all the more promptly. When you figure out how much your association with nourishment can adjust to improve things, you will be charmingly astounded — and this can importantly affect your general prosperity and wellbeing.

Formal dinners, be that as it may, will, in general, assume a lower priority about occupied ways of life for generally people. Rather, supper times are an opportunity to endeavor to do each million stuff in turn. Consider having meals at your work area or accepting your Instagram fix over breakfast to control through a task.

The issue with this is you are bound to be genuinely determined in your decisions about healthy eating and eat excessively on the off chance that you don't focus on the nourishment you devour or the way you eat it.

That is the place mindfulness goes in. You can apply similar plans to a yoga practice straight on your lunch plate". Cautious eating can enable you to tune in to the body's information of what, when, why, and the amount to eat," says Lynn Rossy, Ph.D., essayist of The Mindfulness-Based Eating Solution and the Center for Mindful Eating director.

"Rather than relying upon another person (or an eating routine) to reveal to you how to eat, developing a minding association with your own body can achieve tremendous learning and change."

From the ranch to the fork — can help you conquer enthusiastic eating, make better nourishment choices, and even experience your suppers in a crisp and ideally better way. To make your next dinner mindful, pursue these measures.

The Most Effective Method to Start Eating More Intentionally

Stage 1: Eat Before You Shop. We have all been there. You go with a rumbling stomach to the shop. You meander the passageways, and out of the blue, those power bars and microwaveable suppers start to look truly enticing. "When you're excessively ravenous, shopping will, in general, shut us off from our progressively talented goals of eating in a way that searches useful for the body," says Dr. Rossy. So, even if you feel the slightest craving or urge to eat, get a nutritious bite or a light meal before heading out. That way, your food choices will be made intentionally when you shop, as opposed to propelled by craving or an unexpected sugar crash in the blood.

Stage 2: Make Conscious Food Choices. When you truly start considering where your nourishment originates from, you're bound to pick sustenance that is better for you, the earth, and the people occupied with the expanding procedure portrays Meredith Klein, an astute cooking educator, and Pranaful's author. "When you're in the supermarket, focus on the nourishment source," Klein shows. "Hope to check whether it's something that has been created in this country or abroad and endeavors to know about pesticides that may have been exposed to or presented to people who were developing nourishment." If you can, make successive adventures to your neighborhood ranchers advertise, where most sustenance is developed locally, she recommends.

Stage 3: Enjoy the Preparation Process. "When you get ready sustenance, instead of looking at it as an errand or something you need to hustle through, value the process. You can take a great deal of pleasure in food shopping for items that you know will help you feel better and nourish your body.

Stage 4: "Simply eat". This is something we once in a while do, as simple as it sounds, "simply eat." "Individuals regularly eat while doing different things — taking a gander at their telephones, TVs, PCs, and books, and mingling," claims Dr. Rossy. "While cautious eating can happen when you're doing other stuff, endeavor to' simply eat' at whatever point plausible." She includes that centering the nourishment you're eating without preoccupation can make you mindful of flavors you may never have taken note of. Yum!

Stage 5: Down Your Utensils. When you are done eating, immediately put your dishes and utensils away. This is a way of signaling to yourself that you are done eating (it tends to be much a bit tough to accept). "You're getting a charge out of each chomp that way, and you're focused on the nibble that is in your mouth right now as opposed to setting up the following one," Klein says.

Stage 6: Chew, Chew, Chew Your Food. Biting your sustenance is exceptionally fundamental and not only for, you know, not to stun. "When we cautiously eat our sustenance, we help the body digest the nourishment all the more effectively and meet a greater amount of our dietary needs," says Dr. Rossy. Furthermore, no, we won't educate you how often you've eaten your sustenance. However, Dr. Rossy demonstrates biting until the nourishment is very much separated – which will most likely take more than a couple of quick eats.

Stage 7: Check-In With Your Hunger. You frequently miss the sign that your body sends you during the supper when you eat thoughtlessly, for example, when supper time turns into your prime time to make up for lost time with Netflix appears or when you have your supper in a rush. At the end of the day, the one that illuminates you when you begin to feel total. Dr. Rossy proposes ending dinner and taking some time with your craving levels to check-in. "Keep eating in case no doubt about it," she proposes. "In case you're not ravenous yet, spare the nourishment for some other time, manure it, or even discard it." Those remains can make the following day an incredible dinner of care.

Last but not least, we get it; life does not always allow sit-down, completely tuned-in mealtimes. So if you don't have time for all seven steps, attempt to include one or two in each dinner. "If you have only a little window of time, just try to devote yourself to food," suggests Klein. "Set down your phone, get away from the screen, just be there–you can do that regardless of how much time you have."

Tips in Mindful Eating that Transform how you Relate to Food. We lose ourselves in regular daily existence designs each day. Our propensity vitality pushes and pulls us to and from, and we are left with minimal opportunity to encounter life in a way that, for this very time, we are completely present.

Sometime in the not so distant future, to-day tasks get more from this autopilot state than others. There are a few things we do so regularly in our lives that we become like automatons, doing them all day every day thoughtlessly and commonly. These exercises incorporate strolling, driving, specific sorts of occupation, and (among others) eating.

Yet, these exercises additionally loan themselves to the activity of care, because while these examples are speaking to the draw of propensity vitality, they are likewise the perfect thing to snatch on when in any predefined time we need to turn out to be completely present in our life.

Consideration is both the quality and the activity of getting to be (and remaining) completely present at this very time in our life. It's mindfulness that empowers us to break these standard examples and make a move for a progressively alert and present life.

Eating might be more than whatever another movement that fits the activity of cognizance. This because we discover the flavors we experience when we frequently devour fascinating and various just as the pleasurable demonstration of eating. Thus, it is through the simple exercise of careful gobbling that we can wake up to our life and discover more harmony and joy all the while.

On occasion, we can likewise identify poor practices with nourishment and eating. These poor propensities can cause us a ton of torment, some even respected issue.

The act of eating mindfully can spark a light on our standard eating and sustenance related propensities. What's more, in doing as such, we can ease a lot of the agony on our plate identified with the nourishment.

- **Simply eat mindfully.** Take a minute before eating to see the nourishment's smell, visual intrigue, and even surface. Appreciate the various vibes that go with your feast. This concise minute will help open up your cognizance with the goal that you become all the more completely dynamic in the eating demonstration.

- **Take your time**. Remember to lift your hand/fork/spoon and bite the sustenance itself. Give close consideration to each flavor in your mouth and notice how the nourishment you eat feels and scents. Be completely present for the biting go about as your central matter of (light) focus during cautious eating.

- **Recognize thoughts, feelings, and sensations**. When in your general vicinity of awareness, thoughts, feelings, or different sensations emerge, just be aware of them, recognize their reality, and after that, let them go as though they were gliding on a cloud.

- **Eat (once more)**. Then give back your concentration to the biting demonstration. In the beginning, you will continually lose your mindfulness. Try not to stress; this is typical for any sort of activity of good faith. Simply rehash the procedure from stages 2-4 and attempt to eat mindfully for however much as could be expected of your supper.

- **Pay attention**. While eating mindfully, stay open to any idea, feeling, or feeling that goes into your cognizance field and doesn't attempt to push it away. Acknowledge freely whatever happens, and after that, reclaim your core interest.

The act of eating mindfully is simple. However, there are numerous little tips and deceives that you can take advantage of to help upgrade your ability to eat mindfully and proceed with your routine with regards to mindfulness.

Chapter 15
Learning To Avoid Temptations And Triggers

While telling a person to adopt the traits of the mentally strong is a good way to develop mental toughness, it may not always be enough. In a way it's a bit like telling a person that in order to be healthy you need to eat right, exercise, and get plenty of rest. Such advice is good and even correct, however it lacks a certain specificity that can leave a person feeling unsure of exactly what to do. Fortunately, there are several practices that can create a clear plan of how to achieve mental toughness. These practices are like the actual recipes and exercises needed in order to eat right and get plenty of exercise. By adopting these practices into your daily routine, you will begin to develop mental toughness in everything you do and in every environment you find yourself in.

Keep your emotions in check

The most important thing you can do in the quest for developing mental toughness is to keep your emotions in check. People who fail to take control of their emotions allow their emotions to control them. More often than not, this takes the form of people who are driven by rage, fear, or both. Whenever a person allows their emotions to control them, they allow their emotions to control their decisions, words, and actions. However, when you keep your emotions in check, you take control of your decisions, words, and actions, thereby taking control of your life overall.

In order to keep your emotions in check you have to learn to allow your emotions to subside before reacting to a situation. Therefore, instead of speaking when you are angry, or making a decision when you are frustrated, take a few minutes to allow your emotions to settle down. Take a moment to simply sit down, breathe deeply, and allow your energies to restore balance. Only when you feel calm and in control should you make your decision, speak your mind, or take any action.

Practice detachment

Another critical element for mental toughness is what is known as detachment. This is when you remove yourself emotionally from the particular situation that is going on around you. Even if the situation affects you directly, remaining detached is a very positive thing. The biggest benefit of detachment is that it prevents an emotional response to the situation at hand. This is particularly helpful when things are not going according to plan.

Practicing detachment requires a great deal of effort at first. After all, most people are programmed to feel emotionally attached to the events going on around them at any given time. One of the best ways to practice detachment is to tell yourself that the situation isn't permanent. What causes a person to feel fear and frustration when faced with a negative situation is that they feel the situation is permanent. When you realize that even the worst events are temporary, you avoid the negative emotional response they can create.

Another way to become detached is to determine the reason you feel attached to the situation in the first place. In the case that someone is saying or doing something to hurt your feelings understand that their words and actions are a reflection of them, not you. As long as you don't feed into their negativity you won't experience the pain they are trying to cause. This is true for anything you experience. By not feeding a negative situation or event with negative emotions you prevent that situation from connecting to you. This allows you to exist within a negative event without being affected by it.

Accept what is beyond your control

Acceptance is one of the cornerstones of mental toughness. This can take the form of accepting yourself for who you are and accepting others for who they are, but it can also take the form of accepting what is beyond your control. When you learn to accept the things you can't change, you rewrite how your mind reacts to every situation you encounter. The fact of the matter is that the majority of stress and anxiety felt by the average person is the result of not being able to change certain things. Once you learn to accept those things you can't change, you eliminate all of that harmful stress and anxiety permanently.

While accepting what is beyond your control will take a little practice, it is actually quite easy in nature. The trick is to simply ask yourself if you can do anything at all to change the situation at hand. If the answer is 'no,' simply let it go. Rather than wasting time and energy fretting about what you can't control adopt the mantra "It is what it is." This might seem careless at first, but after a while you will realize that it is a true sign of mental strength. By accepting what is beyond your control, you conserve your energy, thoughts, and time for those things you can affect, thereby making your efforts more effective and worthwhile.

Always be prepared

Another way to build mental toughness is to always be prepared. If you allow life to take you from one event to another you will feel lost, uncertain, and unprepared for the experiences you encounter. However, when you take the time to prepare yourself for what lies ahead, you will develop a sense of being in control of your situation at all times. There are two ways to be prepared, and they are equally important for developing mental toughness.

The first way to be prepared is to prepare your mind at the beginning of each and every day. This takes the form of you taking time in the morning to focus your mind on who you are, what you are capable of, and your outlook on life in general. Whether you refer to this time as mediation, contemplation, or daily affirmations, the basic principle is the same. You simply focus your mind on what you believe and the qualities you aspire to. This will keep you grounded in your ideals throughout the day, helping you to make the right choices regardless of what life throws your way.

The second way to always be prepared is to take the time to prepare yourself for the situation at hand. If you have to give a presentation, make sure to give yourself plenty of time to prepare for it. Go over the information you want to present, choose the materials you want to use, and even take the time to make sure you have the exact clothes you want to wear. When you go into a situation fully prepared, you increase your self-confidence, giving you an added edge. Additionally, you will eliminate the stress and anxiety that results from feeling unprepared.

Take the time to embrace success

One of the problems many negatively-minded people experience is that they never take the time to appreciate success when it comes their way. Sometimes they are too afraid of jinxing that success to actually recognize it. Most of the time, however, they are unable to embrace success because their mindset is simply too negative for such a positive action. Mentally strong people, by contrast, always take the time to embrace the successes that come their way. This serves to build their sense of confidence as well as their feeling of satisfaction with how things are going.

Next time you experience a success of any kind, make sure you take a moment to recognize it. You can make an external statement, such as going out for drinks, treating yourself to a nice lunch, or some similar expression of gratitude. Alternatively, you can simply take a quiet moment to reflect on the success and all the effort that went into making it happen. There is no right or wrong way to embrace success, you just need to find a way that works for you. The trick to embracing success is in not letting it go to your head. Rather than praising your efforts or actions, appreciate the fact that things went well. Also, be sure to appreciate those whose help contributed to your success.

Be happy with what you have

Contentment is another element that is critical for mental toughness. In order to develop contentment, you have to learn how to be happy with what you have. This doesn't mean that you eliminate ambition or the desire to achieve greater success, rather it means that you show gratitude for the positives that currently exist. After all, the only way you will be able to truly appreciate the fulfillment of your dreams is if you can first appreciate your life the way it is.

One example of this is learning to appreciate your job. This is true whether you like your job or not. Even if you hate your job and desperately want to find another one, always take the time to appreciate the fact that you have a job in the first place. The fact is that you could be jobless, which would create all sorts of problems in your life. So, even if you hate your job, learn to appreciate it for what it is. This goes for everything in your life. No matter how good or bad a thing is, always appreciate having it before striving to make a change.

Be happy with who you are

In addition to appreciating what you have you should always be happy with who you are. Again, this doesn't mean that you should settle for who you are and not try to improve your life, rather it means that you should learn to appreciate who you are at every moment. There will always be issues that you want to fix in your life, and things you know you could do better. The problem is that if you focus on the things that are wrong you will always see yourself in a negative light. However, when you learn to appreciate the good parts of your personality, you can pursue self-improvement with a sense of pride, hope, and optimism for who you will become as you begin to fulfill your true potential.

Conclusion

You have learned a lot of things in this guide. You know how to release your anxiety, how to meditate properly, what the most efficient affirmations are. You can do miracles if you use these techniques properly. But pay attention not to overcompensate and not to create another addiction: undereating instead of overeating. Bonnie has fallen into this trap, but as soon as she understood the very root of her problems, she could find her own correct way. Now she is healthy, 54 kilos (119 lbs.) and she has been maintaining her weight for five years. She is married to a smart, generous, loving man. Her husband is not Tony, but her true love! Tony was a wonderful and useful story in her life. Without him, she would have probably never learned to see and appreciate her own real value.

Remember to love your body and your soul, because this is the only way to harmonize them. I wish you a wonderful experience on your way to losing weight!

It does not only help one in weight loss, but it guarantees their general wellbeing. One of the good things about meditation is that you can practice it anywhere and at any time you find convenient. You can also do it at no extra cost. This is a good way to rejuvenate your mind and to focus on the things that matter. It also ensures that you improve your performance levels on the activities that you chose to undertake. With the poor eating decisions that we are making nowadays, we are having increased cases of lifestyle diseases. Obesity is now a huge challenge among the majority of individuals. It is about time that we step up and make better and more informed decisions regarding our lives. Some of these decisions include changing our eating habits and ensuring that we take good care of our health. Meditation helps us to maintain discipline in that which we do. It ensures that we stay focused on the plans and decisions that we have chosen to make. With the right attitude, meditation can transform your weight loss journey.

If you wish to lose weight or maintain a healthy body, you can begin your meditation journey. It is an easy process that you can easily follow up as long as you are determined. All you need to do is decide to start. The journey of a thousand miles begins with a single step. At times you have to go past tapping the waters and get in it completely. In the beginning, you might find it challenging to do so, but it's the encouragement that you keep giving yourself that will ensure you manage to utilize meditation in your weight loss journey successfully.

GUIDED MEDITATIONS FOR ANXIETY

MINDFULNESS MEDITATION
AND SELF-HYPNOSIS EXERCISES
TO MANAGE YOUR EMOTIONS,
STOP WORRYING AND OVERTHINKING, REDUCE STRESS,
OVERCOME PANIC ATTACKS, FIND PEACE AND RELAX

Awakening Transformation Academy

Table of Contents

Introduction

Anxiety is a subjective, complicated emotion. Anxiety is brought by many causes and expressed by a wide range of symptoms. These symptoms may encompass behavioral, cognitive, and emotional components. This is the reason why you can ask a group of individuals about their experience and understanding of anxiety, and get various explanations and definitions which are different from what it means to them to be anxious to them.

People differ in how frequently, and with which intensity, they experience anxiety. The duration over which they have anxiety also differs from one person to another. Most people consider anxiety to be normal, and they have learned to adapt to it when it occurs. An ordinary degree of anxiety is part of our daily human experience. Unfortunately, other individuals experience anxiety to such a heightened level that it leads to great distress. This level of anxiety can impair a person's wellbeing and normal functioning. It can affect several vital areas of a person's life, such as their occupation, studies, and relationships. When anxiety comes to that level where it begins to be distressing and interferes with a person's wellbeing and normal functioning of an individual, then we start to speak of an anxiety disorder.

Anxiety can make life feel like a nightmare. You always fear the worst, so you are constantly negative. You are sometimes paralyzed by fear, which limits how much you do with your life. Your life is restricted more and more as you become more and more fearful. Sometimes, it can be hard or even impossible to talk to other people or to get in your car and drive when you fear the worst all of the time.

The worst part of anxiety is that other people in your life don't understand it. Therefore, they get frustrated with you. They don't understand why you can't just loosen up and have fun. They don't get why you have meltdowns in the middle of grocery stores or why you voice strange and even bizarre fears. "You're so negative," is one of the criticisms that you may experience. Your loved ones may also wonder why they are not enough to calm you down. "I'm here, so you should feel fine," is something that you might hear from your loved ones.

Don't let the negativity of other people bring you down. You suffer from actual mental illness. There is nothing wrong with your personality and you are not stupid just because you can't automatically shut off your symptoms like a faucet. What you suffer is terrible, and no one can take that away from you. Stop listening to critical people and instead start taking care of yourself.

When your life is affected by anxiety, it is time for a change. You may feel that you are resigned to this difficult life forever, but that is not so. There are numerous coping techniques and even cures for what you feel. This book is one of the best first steps that you can take for yourself. This book will show you how to take control of your thoughts when they run wild and put an end to the crippling fears that rule your existence.

For the past ten years of my life, I have dealt with anxiety. I received the formal diagnosis of General Anxiety Disorder when I was eighteen, but I suspect that I suffered from this disorder starting at a much earlier age. I know how it is to be ruled by fear and to have difficulty enjoying life like other people. I also know how it is to "ruin" relationships because of mental illness. While it has taken me a long while to get control over this disorder, I have learned not to let it rule me. Also, I have learned to stop blaming myself. This is a mental disorder that I suffer, not something that is my choice.

While anxiety is not your fault or your choice, it is also not your slave master. You can gain control over it and prevent it from manifesting and ruining your life. You can stop anxiety in its tracks and live life the way that you choose. You just have to learn how, and this book will show you. Overcoming anxiety is an intense mental and personal process that you should dedicate some time to accomplishing. The rewards will be rich.

I will show you some of the things that I have learned over the years about anxiety so that you can understand your disorder better. I will also show you the many tricks and tips I have learned over the years. From meditation to mindfulness as a skill to loving yourself, I will teach you how to think better to avoid the patterns of thinking that lead to anxiety. Finally, I will share a great supplement with you that will make your anxiety disappear. Called Premium Anxiety Formula, this supplement beats medication because it has no side effects and is not habit-forming or expensive. Plus, it works! By the end of this book, you will have the skills to cope and even cure your anxiety.

Keep in mind that these things take work. You cannot just overcome something crippling like anxiety overnight. However, you really can minimize the effects of anxiety on your life very easily and quickly. Almost immediately you will start to notice results if you employ the methods in this book. Still, some of these things take time. Be patient with yourself and with these techniques. Don't give up just because you do not see immediate results. Eventually, you will become the master of your own mind and heal your anxiety. Until then, expect some work and a few setbacks. It is all part of the normal healing process! Just like learning to ride a bike, you are learning a new skill of healing anxiety. So take your time.

Living life with anxiety and depression can be a true nightmare. But you don't have to live in the nightmare forever. I will show you how to successfully climb out of the hole that you may be trapped in now so that you can live life to the fullest and finally heal yourself. I will show you how to begin healing, while also showing you how to cope with your symptoms in the meantime.

Chapter 1
Anxiety

What is Anxiety?

Anxiety is your body's response to the feeling of fear or uncertainty about what is to come. Some of the symptoms synonymous with fear include:

- Rapid breathing

- Racing heart

- A "burst" of energy

- Butterflies in your stomach

Everyone feels anxious at times; whether it's your first day in school, giving a speech, or going for a job interview, this feeling is quite a regular thing. Anxiety can be a way for our body to keep us safe from harm. For example, imagine you're taking a walk through the forest, and you're dragging your feet because you're tired; however, you see something that looks like a bear or a snake at the corner of your eyes. You will suddenly forget that you're tired and feel a burst of energy that helps you get away from that location.

If you feel anxious about an assignment that is due, anxiety will motivate you and can help you get it done faster than you earlier thoughts. However, when you start feeling anxious about something unusual, then it can be very unhealthy. Unhealthy anxiety is what is known as an anxiety disorder. Any anxiety that impacts on your daily life is a disorder. Rather than have anxiety as a response to danger, the person with a disorder begins to feel anxious in situations that are perfectly normal, like taking a means of public transport or meeting new people.

The Negative Effects of Anxiety

Anxiety increases your heart rate and breathing in the short term; it directs blood flow to your brain where it's needed, and this physical response helps you to face an unwanted situation. However, if it gets too intense, it can make you feel nauseous and lightheaded. If anxiety becomes excessive and persistent, it can have a devastating effect on both your mental and physical health.

You can have an anxiety disorder at any point in your life. The symptoms of anxiety can stay hidden for a while, as such; don't wait till you get the sign before you embrace a lifestyle change, start immediately.

Anxiety disorder will affect your:

Central Nervous System

If you've had long-term anxiety and a series of panic attacks, it will make your brain release stress hormones more regularly than it should. This can increase the occurrence of some symptoms, such as dizziness, headaches, and depression. Some hormones and chemicals in your body are designed to help you cope with anxiety when you feel anxious your brain floods your nervous system with these chemicals and hormones. Examples of these chemicals are cortisol and adrenaline.

Excretory and Digestive systems

This might seem too extreme, but it's true. Anxiety has a way of affecting your excretory and digestive systems. Some of the symptoms you'll notice are diarrhea, stomachaches, nausea, and some other digestive issues. You can also experience loss of appetite occasionally.

Some connection has been noticed to exist between the development of irritable bowel syndrome (IBS) after a bowel infection and anxiety. IBS can lead to constipation, vomiting, or diarrhea.

Immune System

Anxiety triggers your flight or fight stress response, which causes a flow of hormones and chemicals like adrenaline into your body system.

This influx of chemicals will increase your breathing and pulse rate so your brain can get more oxygen. This flow of chemicals and hormones prepares you to react well to an intense situation. It can make your immune system function better for a short while. Your body should come back to normal when you are in a calm environment. However, if you regularly feel anxious or the intense situation lasts for a long time, your body never gets the sign to go back to its original state. If your body does not return to its original state, it can weaken your immune system, thus leaving you vulnerable to all types of infections. Your regular vaccines may also not work well if you have an anxiety disorder.

Respiratory System

Anxiety can make you breathe rapidly and shallowly. If you have been diagnosed with chronic obstructive pulmonary disease (COPD), anxiety can land you in the hospital due to anxiety-related complications. Anxiety can also make symptoms of asthma worse.

A Summary of Causes and treatments

Most people feel anxious at some point in their life, but there can be certain factors or triggers that cause other people to feel it more severely than normal. These can include someone's genetics, their environment, how their brain is wired, and what life experiences they've had. If a person associates something with fear, it is likely they will develop anxiety surrounding that thing. Although it is typical for people to have some sort of trigger for their anxiety, this is not true for all cases. Some people have very generalized anxiety about nothing in particular; they are simply always worried or dreading being out in the world.

For some people, one type of anxiety can cause them to develop another type of anxiety. For example, someone who has anxiety about suffering harm or getting sick might develop a germ-related obsessive-compulsive disorder as a way to ensure they will never get sick. Or, people with a social anxiety disorder might eventually develop agoraphobia if they never force themselves to interact with others.

Risk factors for different types of anxiety disorders typically coexist in people who suffer from them, which demonstrates that no single experience is likely to cause someone to develop a disorder. Scientists have found that nature and nurture are strongly linked when it comes to the likelihood that someone will develop severe anxiety. Genetically, research has shown that people have about a 30 to 67 percent chance of inheriting anxiety from their parents (Carter, n.d.). Although someone's DNA might be a factor in them developing anxiety, it cannot account for all of the reasons that have developed it.

Environmental factors should also be taken into consideration when trying to find the root cause of anxiety. Parenting style can be a large factor in whether or not a person will develop anxiety. If parents are controlling of their children or if they model anxious behaviors, the child might grow up thinking these are normal behaviors they should model. This can lead to feeling anxious based on learned behavior. Other factors, such as continual stress, abuse, or loss of a loved one, can also elicit a severe anxious reaction because a person may not know how to handle the situation they find themselves in.

In addition to the environment, a person's health can often cause anxiety as well. If someone is diagnosed or living with a chronic medical condition or a severe illness, it can cause an anxious reaction. One possibility is if the illness is affecting the person's hormones, which can cause stress, or if their feelings of not having control are worsened by a diagnosis they cannot fix.

Some people might not realize that the choices they make daily could be contributing to their anxiety. Things such as excessive caffeine, tobacco use, and not exercising enough can all cause anxiety. Caffeine and other stimulants can increase a person's heart rate and simulate anxiety symptoms. Not exercising can lower a person's level of happy hormones and make their muscles tense or sore, which can also contribute to stress. A person's personality can also

145

determine how severe their anxiety might be. Shy people who tend to stay away from conversations and interaction might develop more severe social anxiety because they are not exposed to those situations often.

When experiencing anxiety, it can seem like there is no way out, but there are actually quite a few different ways a person can work to ease their worries, ranging from clinical to holistic approaches. What type of treatments will work depends on the person, and often, how severe their struggle is.

A few clinical ways to treat anxiety include counseling, psychotherapy, and medication. These are not the only ways a person can be medically treated, but they tend to be the most conventional routes for treating mental illness. Counseling is a type of therapy where the person is able to talk to a licensed practitioner and receive feedback and advice about their situation and how to handle their emotions. Most counselors have a master's degree in the psychology field and are licensed through their state. This type of therapy is usually considered a short-term solution for people who are struggling but not debilitated by their anxiety.

Psychotherapy is typically a more long-term solution for people whose lives are impacted by their anxiety. This type of therapy can focus on a broader range of issues and triggers, such as a person's anxious patterns or behaviors and how to fix them. Cognitive-behavioral therapy is often used in this type of therapy to work with the person to adjust their thoughts and behaviors.

Some people find relief once prescribed medication to help them manage their anxiety. This route is usually reserved for people who are struggling the most and having trouble calming themselves on their own. There are various types of medications, such as SSRIs (selective serotonin reuptake inhibitors) and SNRIs (serotonin-norepinephrine reuptake inhibitors) that alter brain chemicals to reduce anxiety or worry.

Making changes to their lifestyle and habits can also help people with anxiety relieve some of their symptoms. This is a more natural approach to managing anxiety and can be successful for people who are dedicated to making positive life changes. Small things such as diet adjustments and increasing activity levels can reduce anxious feelings. Establishing a consistent sleep schedule is also important to help someone ensure they are getting enough rest each night. Stress fatigues the body, and it may need more time to fully recuperate at night if it was taxed during the day. Making sure the body has a routine can also make someone feel safe and know what to expect from their day.

Meditation can also be a good way for people to calm their minds and ease anxiety. Taking time during the day to be still and quiet might help someone stop the constant worry they feel during the day and relax for a moment. Once they start training their body to relax, it is more likely that they can keep it up during the day. Finally, avoiding stimulants such as caffeine, sugar, and tobacco, and depressants such as alcohol can greatly improve a person's chances of overcoming their anxiety. These substances contribute to the brain's hyperactivity and can often increase feelings of anxiety.

Getting Rid of Anxiety with Meditation

Meditation instructs us to be progressively aware of the

present and less in our minds. We have a propensity for enabling contemplations to enter our psyche and tail them. Occasionally, these are charming considerations, yet commonly these can be stresses, unpleasant musings, on edge emotions, and anxiety.

Frequently, we enable ourselves to pursue these contemplations and even become these considerations. Even though nothing might happen to us physically at that exact second, regardless, we may feel uncertain or on edge about the future because of our reasoning.

Meditation for anxiety is an unmistakable, guided encounter that enables us to work on winding up progressively present, just as furnish a system to manage musings and the truth that is our occupied and dynamic personality. This training is otherwise called care, which once more, prepares our cerebrum to be available by concentrating ceaselessly from intuition and into things that ground us into the present, for example, breathing and physical sensations.

How Anxiety is Reduced with Meditation

Guided meditation for nervousness causes us to watch our contemplations and feelings without decisions. The basic thing the vast majority do when an idea enters their brain is to tail it, judge it, harp on it, and become lost in it. Rather, a standard meditation practice trains us to be available.

This enables us to control the manner in which we see and respond to our nervousness, rather than enabling our uneasiness to control us.

This is supported by studies as well. In fact, Wake Forest Medical Center conducted several of these focusing on brain scans where areas were both deactivated and activated by patients who suffered from anxiety while practicing mindfulness meditation.

It also showed that those volunteers who had no experience with meditation before actually reported relief from anxiety, had their ventromedial prefrontal cortex and anterior cingulate cortex activated. These areas are where both worrying and emotion stem from. Each volunteer had a minimum of 4 sessions that lasted 20 minutes each.

Contemplation for anxiety likewise gives individuals a strategy, instrument to adapt, and arrangement to anxiety and even fits of anxiety as they occur. Frequently, when a fit of anxiety or a wave of anxiety comes, we do not have a clue how to manage it. More often than not, managing it can mean worrying about it, which just serves to intensify the emotions and circumstances. With guided reflection, we have an apparatus that we can go to and use to all the more viably manage anxiety.

Studies have additionally demonstrated that anxiety sufferers who go to guided reflection have revealed expanded sentiments of control, an expanded feeling of general prosperity, just as an expansion in by and large hopefulness. These sentiments go far in alleviating the recurrence and power of anxiety.

Chapter 2
What Is Meditation?

Definitions of meditation vary, but the best one I have seen is: A ritual that allows us to get a good perspective on our lives. Even though it has that effect, meditation is not about becoming a better person per se. When you meditate, you should not be trying to eliminate harmful emotions or bad thoughts. The key is learning how to observe them in an objective manner to get a better understanding (and ultimately, control) of them. Meditation as an activity is a skill that you can only practice but never quite perfect. That is why some people struggle at it while others find it rather easy to do.

Even more important for this book, meditation is the best and most effective way of attaining wellness in all three areas of your life. When you meditate, you attain mindfulness, grounding your mind in the present and eliminating stress. At the same time, your body finds peace during the time of meditation. But it is the specific practices of meditation, like Kundalini Yoga, that really boost our physical wellbeing. Finally, meditating allows us to reconnect with the universe and activate the superconscious mind. The peace that you find from meditating is caused by the fact that by so doing you create the perfect conduit to achieve complete wellness in mind, body, and spirit.

We will discuss meditation in greater depth. We will look at the exact ways through which it boosts out wellbeing in the three key areas of being and energizes us to continue pursuing greatness in everything that we do. We will also look at the exact meditation techniques through which we can enhance our connection to the universe and boost our ability to lead a happy and successful life. But to understand meditation, we have to start from the very beginning and evaluate its origins. Only after understanding the source will we evaluate the exact impact of meditation over our lives and the exact ways to do it.

Why We Meditate

You see, the reason that we meditate is not just because it helps us to improve our concentration span or to end procrastination. These are just the outcomes of meditating. We meditate because it is the only way to connect the physical, intellectual, and spiritual elements of our being. We are made up of the mind, the body, and the spirit.

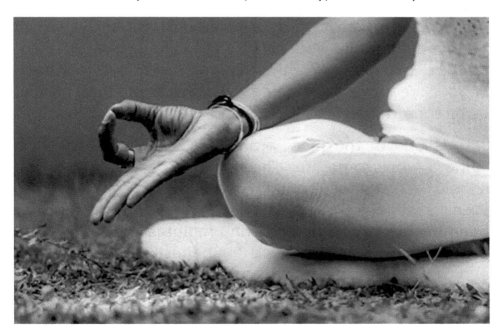

But it is also important to note that the mind is what links the body to the spirit. This is exactly why we meditate. You see, we have the conscious, subconscious, and superconscious minds that correlate with body, mind, and spirit respectively. We meditate to establish a link between all three parts of the brain.

The Conscious

The conscious mind helps us to interpret the world around us. Consciousness is the way we interpret the things we hear, see, touch, smell, and taste. When you manage to activate all these senses (or as many of them as you are able to), then you will be able to achieve a level of mindfulness that allows you to immerse yourself in the present moment. We recognize the conscious mind a lot more than the other levels of the mind because we interact with it a lot more, but it covers the smallest area compared to the other two. Nevertheless, activating your consciousness in everything that you do while you do it will make you a lot more productive. It will give you the chance to live every moment of your life rather than going through the motions without quite appreciating life.

This is one of the most prominent Buddhist lessons on living a wholesome life. The guiding concept is that you should actually be eating while you eat and washing utensils while you wash utensils. And in a world that has been invaded by technology and multitasking, this lesson is even more crucial. It calls for honest self-examination and a willingness to change and live more by overcoming the desire to always be doing as much as possible at the same time.

The Subconscious

The subconscious goes a little deeper than the conscious and touches on our memories and previous life experiences. The subconscious informs our behaviors and reactions to various events by ensuring that all the things we do follow a very specific pattern. This pattern is made of preformed habits, thoughts, and desires. The subconscious has a very interesting relationship with the conscious mind. On the one hand, the conscious mind commands the subconscious reactions that we have to different events. Therefore, if you are confronted by a problem that has previously brought failure into your life, your first reaction will be brought about by your subconscious mind. You will react to that event based on your previous experience with it.

On the other hand, the subconscious mind directs our conscious sensing. This is why you tend to be biased toward certain things or why you love to wear a certain kind of perfume or use a specific type of soap. Your mind has built associations between the things you experience and your feelings. It commands your conscious mind to do certain things to produce a specific kind of effect. Of course, the interaction between the conscious and the unconscious minds is a lot more complicated when you are talking about behaviors that affect success, but the template is the same.

If you want to create real change in your life, you will have to start by working with the subconscious mind to find out why you have experienced failure in your life before. You can then build up a new set of habits and associations in your mind meant specifically to drive you toward success. Meditation is one of the most effective ways to let go of harmful subconscious notions and do some subliminal self-conditioning to attain the highest possible levels of success.

The Superconscious

At the highest level of mindfulness, where most people do not even appreciate its power, is a part of our mind called the superconscious. The superconscious links directly to the god power of the universe—the providence, the infinite power, and the omniscience. You can only activate the superconscious mind for short periods because it is only through meditation that you can do it.

However, when you do activate the superconscious, you will be in a position to reap all the goodness of the universe. Even more notably, it is only through the superconscious that you can discover your life's purpose. This then becomes the driving force of your life and enables you to dedicate your life to something greater than yourself. Being able to reach this level of awareness is one of the key goals of practicing meditation the Buddha way. The connection that you generate between the three levels of consciousness by unlocking the unconscious is basically what nirvana is all about. At this level, you will have the opportunity to harness the power of the universe to manifest great success and prosperity in every area of your life. One important thing to note is that you can only reach this level of awareness through meditation. This is what makes meditation such a critical ingredient in your pursuit of success.

Other Reasons Why We Meditate

Other than the scientific reason for meditation, linking the conscious, subconscious, and superconscious, we meditate to reap the rewards of this practice over our lives.

Meditation Eliminates Stress

Professionals in the most stressful careers can benefit from the stress-relieving benefits of meditation. From teachers to doctors and Wall Street Bankers, meditation has been found to help overcome stress, bring down the levels of depression, and help people overcome burnout (Wanderlust, 2016).

Other than stress, meditation is also the best way to fight anxiety. You see, anxiety has the effect of taking people from the present moment and transporting them into worries about the future. Meditation boosts your brain and helps you to overcome anxiety caused by stressful life events and generalized anxiety disorders.

It Increases Your Level of Happiness

Because meditation helps you to manage your stress in a healthy manner, it gives you a chance to focus on improving your career and relationships. You will even be in a better position to pursue other interests to take the level of your happiness even higher.

Meditation Relaxes You

When you are going through a tough spot, any opportunity to take a break and rewind comes as a godsend. However, the ambitious mind is not designed for relaxation. Even before you are done pursuing your current goal, you will already have a full to-do list of other things that you would like to accomplish. The opportunity to relax with meditation comes in handy because it keeps you grounded and impervious to the small triggers that often unravel the best-made plans.

It Helps Boost Cerebral Activity

Successful people in business, sports, and other areas have been found to have highly integrated brains. These brains improve their functionality and boost their chances of success. Meditation is one of the most effective ways through which you can work to attain this integrated brain functionality and reach success in your chosen field.

Chapter 3
Getting Started

Most people who report having quit meditation also expressed complaints that stem from the lack of understanding of some of these concepts. I, therefore, advise you to read it carefully before proceeding.

We will look into some of the basic ways to start the practice of meditation. We will look at some of the known forms of meditation that would serve as a good starting point, systematically. These are breathing, counting and mindfulness meditation. Remember, if you feel like it might be tricky doing it on your own, you can always seek the assistance of guided meditations and group settings.

The great meditators of the past discovered a connection between external realities and our body and mind. They discovered that we can live a life of higher consciousness by being able to observe what we feel within while still paying attention to without. They discovered that our thoughts and emotions could be our slaves contrary to what is the reality.

To notice how your emotions, shift, observe your breath. When we relax, our breathing is regulated and deep while fast when we experience excitement. With this in mind, the Buddhists discovered that as our breathing can alter our state of mind the same way our state of mind shifts our breathing. In return, this means that if we learn to breathe correctly, we have the power to do away with many unpleasant feelings that torment us on a daily basis.

The negative emotions that we experience coupled with the negative effects they bring about to deal with a lot of damage to our personal and emotional growth. By learning to do away with these self-inflicted vices, we allow ourselves to grow in greater proportions in comparison to people who do not heed this advice. With a calm and clear mind, we make better decisions and play a good fit as a functioning member of society. Before getting into the actual first practice, it would be nice to learn the correct method of breathing.

The natural way our body is supposed to breathe is the abdominal breathing method. At first, it may appear unnatural but this is indeed the natural way for our bodies to breathe. From conception up until a point after birth, this is how our bodies breathe. However, as our age progress, we diverge from this mode of breathing and start breathing while expanding the chest. This newly adopted method only causes the mind to be in a state of anxiety. One should carry out abdominal breathing in this method:

- Assuming you are in a comfortable sitting position, keep an upright posture with your feet apart and touching the ground.

- Place your hands (with the thumbs touching) against the lower section of your belly and let them form a rainbow arc.

- Keeping your chin tucked, press your tongue behind the upper row of teeth. Keep the eyes open and do not stare into any objects.

- Gently, inhale. As you exhale, push out the lower belly and feel the air rush out. Do not completely fill your belly with air; having it three quarters filled is sufficient.

- The exhaling should be equally gentle. It occurs through the nose. Push in your belly to symbolize squeezing out the air. Each step should last you at most 4 seconds each for uniformity.

As aforementioned, it may seem strange to breathe in coordination with the belly for beginners. This gets better and starts to feel more natural with more practice. Furthermore, it is the natural way to breathe.

Beginner Breathing

First, find a good sitting position that will not interfere with the process. You can use the meditation pose or sit on a chair with your hands resting on the sides and a straightened back. Do not get too comfortable though- you might 'meditate' until the next morning.

Minimize any form of distraction that can take your away attention from the meditation process. Some of these things may be a mobile phone, flashing lights, kids looking for your attention, your pet or even the weather. Find out if you should keep warm or wear loose fitted clothes before you start meditating. You may wish to close your eyes or even focus on a specific spot or object in your surroundings.

Once you are seated and comfortable with your eyes closed (or open), relax your muscles and start observing your breath. Do not try to change anything about it. The body knows the amount of air it requires. Just observe your nostrils as air flows naturally through them-in and out. The air may be cool, warm, or itchy. Every feeling is the right feeling- just observe without any judgment.

Stray thoughts may come in droves but do not hate yourself

or form any resentment towards them. Just observe how your mind has the tendency of wandering and try to bring back your thoughts to breathe observation. Keep breathing and keep going deeper. Notice how the sounds around you keep drowning the deeper you take your attention into your breathing.

If stray thoughts keep recurring, notice the pattern of these thoughts. Notice what they are about, what they mostly consist of and if they are from the past or present. Bring your attention back to your breathing and continue observing your breath. At first, it may even be difficult to observe two breaths before the mind wanders. This is totally fine as it is part of the journey. Keep noticing without judgment.

Bodily distractions often come into play when meditating. Some common ones are itching, discomfort or even pain. Sometimes, different sets of emotions may arise such as sorrow or joy but they are impermanent-whatever they are. This should not stop you from the process. Simply observe what they are without judgment and accept whatever stories come up. Then, slowly guide yourself back to observing your breathing.

When your time runs out, bring back your attention to your body and to your surroundings. Notice how relaxed your mind is and how your breath remains the same as you open your eyes. Repeat this daily and cultivate the practice before increasing your time. You are bound to see results.

Mindful Walking Meditation

This technique comes in handy for people who are always on the move or cannot get themselves to sit and meditate. In fact, its efficiency stems from the fact that you do not need to add another routine to your daily activities to make it work. All you have to do is walk mindfully. You can always walk mindfully as you carry on with your normal routine. This practice helps to cultivate a lot of awareness as one observes within while facing the distractions of life.

It would be advisable to choose an appropriate place where you are likely to get fewer distractions as well as have good walking space. Begin with a stationary, upright position. Feel the weight of your body on your feet. You have the freedom to place your hands behind, either resting on your sides or even clasped around your chest- whatever feels comfortable. As you do this, remain relaxed and observe whatever sensations you feel objective.

Start walking using short slow steps and pay attention to the feelings that arise and pass on your feet. These feelings can vary from pain, pressure, heat or even heaviness. There is no right or wrong feeling to experience. All you have to do is observe them as they arise and pass. In this practice, the feelings one encounters as they walk are the anchor unlike in breathing meditation.

Keep walking and pay close attention to the sensations experienced on your feet as you make every step. As your foot rises and as it falls back to the ground, what do you feel? After making nonjudgmental observations, keep walking towards the chosen destination while keeping a natural and relaxed posture. When you get to the end of the walk, stand for a couple of seconds, and observe what your body feels. Before turning, center your attention back to your feet and start walking slowly again.

If the initial pace is chosen does not seem to suit the experience, feel free to switch it up a bit to the level of your comfort. You might find that walking fast works better for you! Notice how impermanent the walk is; how you keep going back and forth in the same path. You may also notice how impermanent the sensations that occur as you walk are. Just simply observe and keep practicing.

In comparison to beginner breathing, the mind is bound to wander even when doing mindful walking. This is totally fine. Noticing that your mind has wandered is half the journey. You, however, need to refocus your attention back to the next step gradually. If you notice your mind spent twenty minutes wandering, that is still fine. The fact that you noticed and refocused yourself is the most important part. Oh, and keep your eyes open!

Counting Meditation

Counting meditation is exactly as it sounds. You just need to be relaxed with your eyes closed and count up to the desired number. Ridiculous? I think not! Do you remember when we talked about the use of anchors? In this case, the numbers are your anchor. Anytime the mind decides to drift away, slowly bring back your attention to where you left off and continue counting. A practice like this can really do wonders for your attention span. Remember to observe with no judgment.

If the real intention is present when performing this practice, you will notice the intensity of the thought patterns subsides. Your thoughts will go in tandem with the counting. The more you learn to bring back your mind to focus, the more your mind detaches itself from its habitual patterns. Self-awareness develops.

These are just some of the basic meditation techniques that serve as great starters for a new meditator. If you grasp either one of these first, transitioning to the rest of the techniques taught in this book will be easy as one, two, and three.

Chapter 4
How To Calm The Body

Exercise is a highly recommended stress reliever for many reasons. Physical activity has many benefits in addition to reducing stress, and these benefits alone (increased health, longevity, and happiness) make exercise a worthwhile habit. And as a stress management technique, it is more effective than others. The combined benefits of these two facts make physical exercise a lifestyle that is worth following.

Do physical activity

The definition of physical activity in this context has not been limited only to exercise. Physical activity is any activity that engages your physique. Mostly it will lead to perspiration. When an individual engages in physical activity, he or she is obliged to concentrate fully on that particular activity. Exercising is a very renowned way to counter depression. Regular exercise has time and again been used as an anti-depressant. When one is exercising, endorphins are boosted. These are chemicals that enable an individual to feel good.

The statistics of how many people deal with stress is always on the upward. When one experiences stress, it has a lasting effect in their lives since it cuts across what an individual is engaging in at a particular time. To eradicate stress completely is an uphill task, and one would rather manage it. Exercising is one of the best methods to manage stress. Many medical practitioners advise that individuals should engage in exercises in a bid to manage stress levels.

The advantages that come with a person engaging in exercises have far been established to be a counter-measure against diseases and as a method of enhancing the body's physical state. Research has it that exercising helps a great deal when decreasing fatigue and enhancing the body's consciousness of the environment. Stress invades the whole of your body, affecting both the body and mind. When this happens, the act of your mind feeling well will be pegged on the act of the body feeling well too. When one is in the act of exercising, the brain produces endorphins that act naturally as pain relievers. They also improve the instances upon which an individual falls asleep. When the body is able to rest, this means that its amounts of anxiety have dropped by a large margin. Production of endorphins can also be triggered by the following practices. They include but are not limited to meditation and breathing deeply. Participation in exercise regularly has proven an overall tension reliever.

Doing relaxation exercises

Another method of reducing stress levels is through the use of some relaxation techniques. A relaxation technique is any procedure that is of aid to an individual when trying to calm down the levels of anxiety. Stress is effectively conquered when the body itself is responding naturally to the stress levels in the body. Relaxation can be often confused with laying on a couch after a hard day. This relaxation is best done in the form of self-meditation, although its effects are not fulfilling on the impact of stress. Most relaxation techniques are done at the convenience of your home with only an app.

The following types of exercise are highly recommended for stress reduction because they have specific properties that are effective in reducing stress in short and long-term stress management:

Yoga

The gentle stretching and balance of yoga may be what people think when they practice, but there are several other aspects of yoga that help reduce stress and to have a healthy life. Yoga entails the same type of diaphragmatic breathing; this is used with meditation. In fact, a few yoga styles include meditation as part of their practice (in fact, most types of yoga can take you to some degree of meditation).

Yoga also includes balance, coordination, stretching, and styles are the exercise of power. All support health and stress reduction. Yoga can be practiced in many ways. Some yoga styles feel like a gentle massage from the inside, while others sweat and hurt you the next day, so there is a yoga school that can work for most people, even for those who have some physical limitations, to be attractive.

Walking

Walking is one of the easiest medications to relieve stress that is excellent because of the benefits this technique offers. The human body was designed to travel long distances, and this activity generally did not cause as much wear as it did. Walking is an exercise that can be easily separated by the speed you use, the weights you carry, the music you listen to, and the location and the company you choose.

This type of exercise can also be easily divided into 10 minutes of sessions, and classes are not needed, and no special equipment is needed beyond a good pair of shoes. (This is an advantage since studies have shown that three 10-minute workouts provide the same benefits as a 30-minute session: great news for those who, due to their busy schedule, need to practice in parts! To find the More smalls!)

Martial Arts

There are many forms of martial arts, and although each one may have little focus, ideology, or set of techniques, they all have benefits to relieve stress. These practices tend to pack both aerobic and strength training, as well as the confidence that comes from physical and self-defense skills.

Generally practiced in groups, martial arts can also offer some of the benefits of social support, as classmates encourage each other and maintain a sense of group interaction. Many martial arts styles provide philosophical views that promote stress management and peaceful life, which you can choose or not accept. However, some styles, especially those with high levels of physical combat, have a higher risk of injury, so martial arts are not for everyone, or at least not all styles work for everyone. If you try several different martial arts programs and talk to your doctor before following the style, you have a better chance of finding a new habit that keeps you fit for decades.

These three examples are not the only types of exercise. They simply show some benefits and are usable by most people. There are many other forms of workout that can be very powerful, such as Pilates, running, weight training, swimming, dancing, and prepared sports.

Everyone brings their stress management benefits to the table, so discover and practice the form of exercise that appeals to you the most.

Mindfulness Body Scan Meditation

This technique requires a more formal atmosphere than the breathing technique as it is best experienced when you are lying down or sitting in a really comfortable posture. While lying down may seem like a fabulous way, initially, it might not be a good idea in the long-run because novices tend to fall asleep in this position. Also, while a good 30-minute duration is needed for effective results, you may make the best use with whatever little time you get.

Sit down on a cushion or a chair or lie down comfortably on the floor. Avoid lying on a mattress if you find it difficult to stay awake. Close your eyes because it makes it easy to focus. Now, pay attention to your breath. Slowly move your attention to the places where your body is in contact with your chair or floor. Investigate each of your body mentally.

The different sensations you experience could be tingling, pressure, tightness, temperature, or anything else. Sometimes, you may not feel any sensation too. Notice the absence of sensations also. Your body becomes an anchor for your mind to hold on so that it doesn't wander away.

Again, be aware when your mind wanders, and gently get it back to where it was before it moved off. When you are done, open your eyes, and mindfully get your focus back on the outside environment.

Another crucial aspect of the body scan mindfulness

technique is to release the tension in the various parts of your body as you scan it. When you focus on a particular section of the body, say your shoulders, you suddenly realize that you are holding them too rigid and creating tension in that area. By focusing on that part, tension is automatically released from there.

These are formal ways of body scans and breathing mindfulness meditation techniques. You can do these mindfulness activities even while sitting in your chair in your office. Take a 5-minute break and do a body scan or focus on your breath even as you sit at your desk. You don't even have to get up from your seat. Also, you could do it during your daily commute or while waiting for someone or standing in line for something or anywhere else. Mindfulness meditation does not need anything else but your mind, which is always with you.

Mindfulness Meditation through Mantra Chanting

A mantra is a phrase, word, or syllable that is repeated during the meditation session. Mantras can be repeated in mind, whispered, or chanted aloud. Mantra meditation involves two elements, including the mantra that is being chanted and mindfulness meditation using the mantra as the anchor. Mantra chanting keeps the mind focused and facilitates mindfulness meditation. People also use the mantra as a form of positive affirmations.

Identify the best mantra for your needs. You can choose your mantra based on the reason for the mantra chanting. Are you looking at getting back your health? Are you seeking peace? Do you desire for something to happen in your life? Are you looking for a deep spiritual awakening?

Sit comfortably with your back straight but not rigidly erect. Focus on your breathing first, which will help you get into the mindfulness meditation state. Ensure your intention for the mantra chanting and meditation is clearly imbibed in your mind. Now, start chanting the mantra. Don't expect miracles when you start your chant. Simply repeat the mantra slowly, deliberately, and in a relaxed manner. In this mindfulness meditation technique, mantras are the anchors that help your mind to focus.

There are no 'best' mantras for mindfulness meditation. You can choose anything from the scriptures of your personal religion, or you can choose positive and empowering affirmations such as:

- I am happy and content at this moment.

- All my treasures are inside of me.

- My heart is my best guide.

- Its always now.

- I am complete, and I don't need anything outside of me to make me whole.

- Nothing is permanent.

- This too shall pass.

Chapter 5
Breathing Exercises Throughout the Day

Breathing is a fundamental principle of our lives. You must breathe in and out to live. Many times, people suffer from breathing-related problems, which later on affect them. Some have lost their dear lives because of having difficulties in breathing. Others are suffering because they are unable to breathe well. Therefore, it is essential to note the exact significance of breath.

The first important of breathing is that it reduces anxiety. Breathing also helps in the elimination of insomnia. It has the power to manage your day to day cravings, and also it can control and manage your anger response. Breathing brings your whole body into more excellent balance as it can initiate calmness within you. You will realize your entire being becomes normal again after a proper process of breathing and level of stress will be no more. For those having a high level of emotional frustrations can also apply breathing techniques all through the day so that they might get well too. Nothing is as sweet and pleasant as having an excellent relaxed body.

Breathing also aids in other functions within your bodies, such as muscle relaxation, digestion, and even peristalsis processes. The movement of fluids within your body is made possible by the help of breathing. Breathing helps in the transportation of your body elements such as nutrients and oxygen. It also aids in the removal of waste products. It is better to note that breathing has got that most considerable impact on your respiration as it can donate the required oxygen for respiration. You can acquire the exact energy needed for normal body functions. You will feel strong because power has been formed in your body tissue. Your muscles will be stable since the energy to undertake all your body functions are there. Therefore, you will realize that breathing is a continuous and dynamic process that has no end. Throughout the day, you will understand that breath is an incurring process. We are going to look at several breathing ways that can help eliminate and reduce any form of anxiety within you.

The first breathing technique that you will realize is part and parcel of your whole day is reducing stress through breathing. Before doing this breathing process, try as much as possible to adopt a good sitting position. The position should be comfortable and relaxing. You can also place your tongue behind your front upper teeth and do the following:

- Start by making sure your lungs are empty. You can do this by allowing the air inside to escape through your nose and mouth. You can facilitate this process by doing some enlargement of your shoulder and chest and contracting your stomach so that you increase the exhale process.

- Now you can breathe in through your nose. It should be tranquil and silent. Remember, it is supposed to take only 4 seconds.

- The next step is to hold your breath, let's say for about 7 seconds. Don't rush here as your breath should just come naturally.

- Then go ahead by breathing out. You have to force all air out through your mouth. You can purse your lips too and making some sounds of your preference. This should take at least 8 seconds.

- Repeat this process four times.

Therefore, this breathing technique to delete stress in life is seen as a formidable way to control anxiety. Many researchers, such as Dr. Weil, have recommended these techniques to many patients of anxiety they have healed. According to him, you need to do it in four cycles so that you start realizing its benefits. He went ahead by illustrating that, the moment you do this, feeling of lightheaded encroaches. This will help you to feel relaxed and calm. A relaxed mind and feeling of calmness clear off the stress in your mind. Therefore, your level of anxiety will reduce. You will start having a perfect life without stress and anxiety. Remember, this process takes time. It is now recommended that you perform it in a sitting position that's not only affordable but also comfortable. This type of breathing is the famous 4-7-8 breathing.

The next breathing technique that you can efficiently perform is belly breathing. Belly breathing is not difficult to implement. It is among the most straightforward breathing techniques that can eventually help you to release stress. The following steps are deemed appropriate for your breathing.

- Look for a sitting posture or lie flat in any way as far as it is comfortable.

- Place your hands on both your belly and chest, respectively. Remember to put one and just below the rib cage.

- Now you can start breathing. Take an intense breath through your nose and let your hand be pushed out of its position by the belly. The other hand should not move even an inch.

- The next step is to breathe out very loud and produce that whistling sound with your pursed lips. You can feel that palm on your belly moves in as it pushes out the air.

- You are allowed to repeat this process more than ten times and make sure to take your time with every single breathing you are undertaking.

- Remember to make a note on your feelings at the end of the whole process.

Therefore, belly breathing is a type of breathing that will help you to reduce tension within your stomach tissues. Your chest tissues and even your ribs will feel relaxed. In the end, the anxiety within your body decreases, and your calmness comes back to normal.

We also have roll breathing that you can eventually use to delete some sorts of anxiety, stress, depression, and even unpleasant feeling within you. Roll breathing has several important in your body. Roll breathing enlarges your lungs and, as a result, makes you be able to pay a close watch on your breathing. The rhyming and rhythm of your breath become your full focus. You can undertake this breathing anytime and anywhere. However, as a learner, you should use your back on the ground with your legs bent. Then start by doing the following:

- Place your two hands on your belly and chest, respectively. Take a note on the movement of your hands as you concentrate on your breathing process. Continue breathing in and out.

- Focus on filling the lower lungs so that your belly moves up when you are inhaling while your chest does not move an inch. It is better to note that breathing in should be through your nose while breathing out must be through your mouth. You are allowed to repeat this process even ten times so that you can realize better results.

- After filling and emptying your lungs, you can now perform the other step of filling your upper chest. You can manage this by first inhaling in your lower lungs then increasing the tempo so that it reaches the chest. Here, you should breathe regularly but slowly for quite sometimes. During this process, note the position of your two hands. One placed at the belly will slightly fall as the stomach contract. The one put on your chest will rise as more air is breathed in your chest.

- It is now your time to exhale. Go ahead by exhaling slowly through your mouth. You should make that whooshing sound when your hands start falling, respectively. Always, your left hand will have to fall first, followed by your right hand. Still, on this, notice the way tension leaves your body as your mind becomes relaxed and calmed.

- Repeat the whole process of breathing in and out for at least 3 to 5 minutes. In this case, make sure you are observing the movement of your chest and belly. Take note of the rolling waves motion.

- Your feeling matters a lot in the whole process. Take a more exceptional look at how you feel in the entire rolling breathing.

Your body regains its full free state, and you will feel more relaxed. You can, therefore, practice this rolling breathing process daily and make sure this goes for several weeks. By doing so, you will be able to perform this kind of breathing exercise everywhere. Also, you can eventually achieve this instantly on most occasions. It will help you regain your relaxation and calmness back. At the end of rolling breathing, your anxiety will be at bay. However, this process is not for everyone since some may feel dizzy during the exercise. You can reduce the breathing speed and accelerate slowly. You can then get up slowly after feeling relaxed, calmed, and lightheaded.

Another breathing technique is morning breathing. When you wake up, your body is still exhausted and tired. You feel that your muscles are still weak and wholly tensed. You will realize that your stiffness has got an impact on your day to day activities. The best breathing exercise to follow here is the morning breathing process. It can clear any clogged breathing passages. You can use this method throughout the day to remove the back tension that may be a nagging and a worrying issue to you. The following steps will eventually help you to perform this task with much ease and less effort.

- Stand still and then try to bend forward. You should slightly bend your knees, and your hands should closely dangle on the floor or close to it.

- Start inhaling and slowly exhaling, followed by a deep breath as you return into a standing position. You can roll upward slowly and making sure that your head comes last from the ground.

- Take your time and hold your breath, whether for five seconds or even for 10 seconds. You should do this in your standing position.

- Start exhaling. That is, breathing out slowly while trying to make a return to your initial position. You can bend forward a little bit.

- Take note of your feelings at the end of the exercise.

The most important thing about this breathing exercise is that it has the power to instill in you more energy, thus enabling you to carry on with every task of the day. You will be relaxed and calm. The level of anxiousness will reduce. In the end, you will feel more lightheaded and entirely energetic.

The next breathing exercise throughout the day can also involve skull shining breath. The skull shining breath is also known as kapalabhati in another language where the term initially originated. It is a dominant type of breathing that enables you to acquire a relaxed and calm mind and brain. It always boasts of the right way of killing the anxiety in you by eliminating the tension, especially in your skull. Remember, it is good to note that the pressure of the head can negatively influence your whole day, and the impact can remain with you for long.

Skull shining breath is not difficult to undertake, and this will give you that morale of even performing it throughout the day. You can start by having long breathing in then follow it with a quick and extremely powerful breathing out. Exhaling should originate from your belly, especially the lower part.

However, after getting familiarized with the whole contraction process, you can now start on inhaling and exhaling at a faster rate. Increase your pace here and make sure all the breathing process takes place through the nose. In this process, do not involve your mouth at the initial stages. You can go on with the process repeatedly until you start feeling very much relaxed.

You can now take note of your feelings at the end of the breathing exercise. Remember, this breathing process can eventually prevent muscle tension too. It also helps in releasing abdominal pain. Your worries, stress, anxiety, and even clogged breathing sites will be well.

Breathe Deep

Throughout any day, there are bound to be things that cause your stress levels to rise slightly. There are also going to be thoughts that pop into your head and cause you to feel anxious. Our mind can be our own worst enemy, but the good news is we can take control. There are many ways that we can help ease our fears, and deep breathing is one of them!

These techniques are extremely easy to do and can be done anywhere, even at your desk or on the bus to work! If you find it hard to concentrate, you can also purchase a guided relaxation tape, or download a stress-relieving app, as these will guide you through breathing exercises until you get the hang of doing them yourself.

Try this:

- Close your eyes and breathe in through your nose for a count of five, hold it for five, and then exhale through your mouth for five, in a slow and controlled manner. Repeat that for as long as you need to gain control.

- Once youre feeling a little calmer or in control, picture the thing that is causing you stress or anxiety as an item or a color. For instance, it might be a black ball, or it might be a gray cloud. It doesnt matter what it is; it simply needs to symbolize the thing that is negatively affecting your day.

- Now, visualize yourself forcefully pushing that item far away from you, and visualize it disappearing into the distance.

- Finish off with the same breathing technique you started with, before gently coming back into the room.

This is a method you can use for any type of stress or anxiety that is bothering you, and it's a great way to get rid of an issue that is upsetting you at any stage during the day.

Another essential breathing technique is ensuring that we are taking deep, full breaths. When we are even the slightest bit stressed, we start breathing shallowly. These shallow, short breaths do not give us enough oxygen and can even lead to full-blown panic attacks. To stop poor breathing, place your hand an inch or two above your stomach. Now, slowly breathe in through your nose until your stomach touches your hand. Go with our usual 5 counts inhales, and hold for a few seconds before slowly exhaling out through your mouth.

When our breathing is shallow, we only fill up the top portion of our lungs with air. Placing your hand above your stomach ensures that you are breathing deeply enough where your entire lungs are filled!

Deep breathing is the foundation of many calming strategies. It can be done on its own or with other methods like meditation, tai chi yoga, etc. Deep breathing is easy because we need to breathe to remain alive, but strongly and efficiently for mental relaxation and stress reduction. Deep breathing focuses on breathing the stomach thoroughly and clean singly. It is easy to learn that you can do it anywhere, and it regulates your stress levels. Sit down with your back straight, inhale through the nose as the belly grows. Inhale as much clean air as possible into the lungs. It makes it possible to get more oxygen into the blood. Exhale the mouth as the belly drops to force as much air as possible out and close the abdominal tract. If you find it difficult to do this sitting, first try to lie down. You could put your hands on your chest and stomach to see if it's wrong.

Chapter 6
Meditation for Anxiety

Throughout this book, we have taken the time to understand anxiety, its triggers, signs, and some of the types of anxiety disorders. It has become clear that everyone faces anxiety at one point in their lives while others seem to have it constantly haunting them. It also became clear how the word does not get the recognition it deserves.

We are going to look into different meditation techniques which are used to deal with anxiety and panic disorders. If you are suffering from either, this is the book for you. Who knows, it might save you the frequent trips to the doctor to get anxiety pills.

Anxiety and Stress Relief

The goal of anxiety and stress relief meditation is to learn how to let go of whatever is weighing you down and realize the peace and calmness the mind can experience. It serves the purpose of helping someone understand the position they are now in. The past and the future are impermanent. By letting these thoughts cloud our judgment and state of mind, we accept the troubles they drag along with them.

When it comes to anxiety and stress relief, it is highly advisable to separate yourself from everyone else. You need time to restore yourself to your most productive element because you might rub off some of the bad energy onto others. If need be, hide in a properly ventilated closet-as long as you are comfortable.

Close your eyes and try to relax your body. This is important to prepare it to get into a state of well-being. Focus your attention on yourself. This is your time; forget all the other things that cloud your mind. You want to be at peace and resonate peace and this is your time to manifest its existence. Start by inhaling and exhaling slowly through the nose and mouth in that order. Observe your body and the buildup of tension accumulated from the anxiety and stress.

You can imagine a stream of river passing and washing away all the buildup of anxiety and stress. Let it all go; let it all wash away. You can imagine anything. You can also decide to fold your stress and anxiety in a leaf and let it go in whichever direction the wind decides. Every time you exhale, envision all the worries go away. Your mind is your palace of imagination. You can do anything in the space you have created for yourself now.

Slowly, go back and observe your breathing again. Keep inhaling through your nose and exhaling through the mouth. You can decide to let it happen naturally or give it intervals of three seconds. Your space your choice. If your mind keeps wandering, you can perform a couple of deep breaths to bring back your focus to your breathing.

Now, imagine you are all alone at the beach and you have worn your favorite pair of swimsuits. You want to take a dip because you are aware of the calming effect water has on you. Picture yourself running towards the water and splashing your way in. To your surprise, when you take a dip, you start to glow and feel so nice. The more you dip yourself into the water, the more your worries wash away leaving you with a nice aura and a sense of peace. Keep imagining this before going back to observe your breathing.

Notice if there is any change in your breathing. Does it feel more natural and relaxed? Do you feel better? If not, start with the breathing again. Center yourself and your thoughts. Do not let your source of stress or anxiety plague you in this space. Remember, this is your personal space. This is your time. Nobody can take away your time.

You can use any relevant scenario as a visual tool to let go of the stress and anxiety that had manifested itself. It does not have to be exactly what is above. If it works for you, that is all that matters. Keep transitioning from your breathing to visual scenarios until the time you desire. Even after feeling better, you might decide to continue doing it for a while just because you can. There is certainly no harm in that.

Apart from the above method, mindfulness meditation, some audio guided meditations and Vipassana meditation serve as good alternatives to try. The practice of meditation does not restrict you from trying out something different if the one you are accustomed to doing does not show results. Any technique that is good for you is the best.

Self-Healing for On-The-Spot Anxiety

Anxiety can clock in at any time it feels like. Let us compare it to that manager who decides to walk into the office, yet nobody expected them to show up because it was their day off. From minor misunderstandings to large problems, anxiety always comes packed differently to every individual. Luckily, several methods that deal with anxiety immediately occur exist. These methods are:

Mindful Breathing

Take some time out for yourself for just five minutes. If you cannot, just pay attention to yourself wherever you are and start to breathe deeply while assuming an upright posture. Notice how the lower section of your bells expands as you breathe in through your nose and contracts as you breathe out through your mouth. Deep breathing is associated with lowering the heart rate, which in turn reduced blood pressure.

Focus on the Present

As soon as you feel the anxiety starting to kick in, in whatever situation you are, just start to focus on what is happening presently. If you are walking, focus on how your feet hit the ground and how the wind is blowing against your face or hair. If you are eating, focus on how your

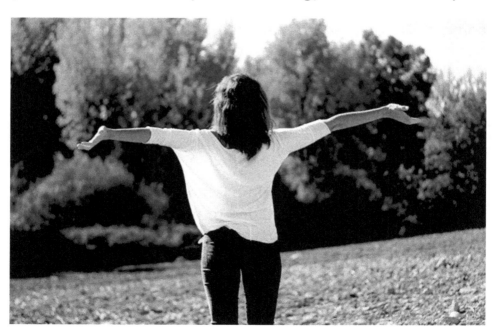

fingers feel holding that spoon. What kind of sensations do you feel around your mouth as you eat? Pay attention to these details and slowly witness yourself starting to feel less tense.

Scan Your Body

This technique combines bodily awareness and breathing. It helps individuals experience the connection between the body and the mind. Start by observing your breathing. Inhale and exhale through your nose. The purpose is to clear all the stories in your head and concentrate on yourself. After a few minutes, focus your attention on a specific group of muscles and release any tension you feel. Move to the next muscle and so the same. Keep doing this until you have covered the whole body. You can do it in whatever order you like.

Use Guided Imagery

Due to the availability of the internet, it is easy to find apps or audios online that can help you create guided images. However, this technique might not be so efficient for people who have a problem constructing mental images. If you have the ability to construct mental images with ease, make sure that the imageries are relatable to you. Otherwise, you might not understand what is going on- which beats the whole point. Guided imageries are there to help someone reinstate the positivity in themselves. If you find it difficult to visualize such images in your mind, you can stare at one imagine for a few seconds, and then close your eyes with the idea of retaining the image in your mind. As you practice this technique, you will find it to be easier and easier to achieve mental imagery.

Start Counting

In school, it was a common thing to hear teachers or parents say, "If you feel angry or you want to say something out of bitterness, just count to ten first." It is funny how this holds true. Counting is one of the many easy ways to deal with your anxiety anywhere it occurs. You do not have to count to ten; you can even do it to one hundred if it feels right. Challenge yourself and count backward as well. This way, you can really get your mind into it.

Sometimes the anxiety goes away quickly, while other times it does not. Whatever the case, ensure you try to keep calm and collected. Counting distracts you from the cause of anxiety and keeps your mind busy. This will eventually return you to a state of calm.

Interrupt Your Thoughts

From my experience with anxiety, your thoughts can so powerful to the extent of making you actually feel like your fears are going to manifest themselves. The thought itself then again doubles your anxiety and the cycle just keeps going. Then again, you realize that the majority of these things never get to happen and that you were so anxious for no good reason.

Interrupting your thoughts as they come can bring you back to a sense of calm. You can do this by starting to think about a person you love- a person who brings peace into your life. If you like a certain music album, skip to your favorite songs and jam along. Remember to always return your focus to yourself and observe how you feel after a few minutes. Observe how none of these feelings is permanent.

With these few tips, you are ready to break your anxiety cycle.

Panic Attacks

A panic attack is an unexpected feeling of intense fear that leads to other serious physical responses where no actual risk or obvious cause is present. They may occur at any time, even when you are asleep. Sometimes they have no trigger. A panic attack gives you breathing difficulties, makes your heart pound and it gives you a feeling that you are going crazy or are about to die. It is not a pretty experience just from what it sounds like. Other symptoms that occur may include sweating, shaking, fever, nausea, your legs may 'turn to jelly' and feeling a disconnection from yourself.

Many people only get to experience less than five panic attacks in their lifetime. The problem usually then goes away after the stressful episode has ended. Some people have very constantly recurring panic attacks and they happen to stay in constant fear with the danger of having another panic attack-these people suffer from a condition called panic disorder.

It is difficult to pinpoint what exactly causes feelings of panic and the onset of attacks, but they tend to be common in families. Major life events such as marriage, graduation and retirement and the death of someone you love also show a bond with panic attacks and panic disorders. Some medical conditions can also be cause panic attacks such as hyperthyroidism and low blood sugar. The use of stimulants in the likes of caffeine and cocaine can also trigger panic attacks and disorders. If you suffer from panic disorders, it would be advisable to refrain from such.

In the event that you have had a panic attack and it has passed, it would be nice to give your body what it needs.

You might feel fatigued, hungry, or even thirsty. Make sure you give yourself some good treatment after it happens. It is advisable to inform someone that you can confide in about the situation. It is not a bad thing to ask for help.

Below are breathing techniques that reverse the symptoms of panic disorders.

Diaphragm Meditation for Panic Attacks

When we encounter a situation of distress, the pattern and rate of our breathing become different. On a normal day, we always breathe slowly using our lower lungs. However, in situations of distress, our breathing shifts to be shallow and rapid while situated in the upper lungs. In the event that it happens when resting, it can cause hyperventilation. This also explains some of the symptoms experienced during panic. Luckily, by knowing how to change your breathing, you can start to reverse the symptoms of your panic attack.

The body has a natural calming response called the parasympathetic response that triggers by changing how you breathe. It is very powerful and is the complete opposite of the emergency response (the feelings that kick in during an attack). When the calming response comes into play, all the primary changes brought about by the emergency response start to shift.

The two meditation techniques recommended to help with this disorder are natural breathing technique and the calming counting technique. The natural breathing technique is pretty much the same thing as the abdominal breathing technique. If you can practice breathing like this on a daily basis, it will only prove beneficial.

The Natural Breathing Technique
(Abdominal Breathing Method)

Gently inhale a normal amount of air through your nostrils making sure it fills your lower lungs. You can decide to place your hands beneath your lower belly to supervise this or you can do whatever seems comfortable. Make sure to exhale easily while focusing on the movements of your lower belly. Feel it expand as air gets in and go down when you exhale. Carry this practice with a relaxed mindset not forgetting to fill your lower lungs with air. Try your best to actually "feel" the oxygen rushing into your body and making its way through your blood. You will feel how every tissue in your body imbibes the fresh oxygen you have just inhaled.

Calming Counts

Assume a comfortable sitting posture and take a deep breath. As you are exhaling, slowly whisper to yourself to relax. Keep your eyes closed to avoid losing focus. Now, start taking natural breaths while counting down from a desired number. Make sure to only count after a successful exhale. As you keep breathing, throw your attention to any areas of tension. Imagine the tension getting loose and shriveling, leaving you feeling calm and refreshed.

When you arrive at the end of your countdown, open your eyes, and notice any difference in what you are feeling. If it has worked but not as efficiently as desired, give it a longer try making sure your willpower is set to let go of the panic. Eventually, you will notice yourself get better.

Studies have shown that these meditation techniques, if practiced even when one is not anxious, are bound to yield the same results. If you can, dedicate a little time every morning and evening to practice the technique that works best for you.

Two things should be highly observed when practicing these techniques: focusing on changing negative thoughts and not thinking of anything else while meditating. This is because our thoughts directly influence our breathing and changing your negative thoughts can help lessen the symptoms quickly. Concentrate most of your effort into not thinking about anything else. Do not even think about your next breath; it should happen naturally.

Chapter 7
Guided Meditation for Anxiety

Find a comfortable place to sit. Either on a chair or on the ground.

Adjust your posture accordingly and sit upright with your spine straight, neck tall and shoulders relaxed.

When you are ready, gently close your eyes.

Allow yourself to settle in the here and now.

(10 seconds)

Become aware of your surroundings. Notice any sounds around you. They may be loud or subtle. Maybe there is a sound of the clock ticking. Or, the humming noise of your air conditioning. Or, noise from the streets. Maybe you can hear the chirping of the birds outside. Or, it is completely silent. Just notice whatever sounds or silence in your environment.

(20 seconds)

Now, pay attention to your thoughts and notice what thoughts are popping up in your mind

(5 seconds)

What are you thinking about?

Are you thinking of your problems or your plans for the day?

Just become aware of the thoughts in your mind and let them go.

(10 seconds)

Now, bring your attention to your breathing.

Take a deep breath in through your nose and feel it fill your body.

(5 seconds)

Exhale completely and let the air leave your body.

(5 seconds)

Keep breathing deeply.

(30 seconds)

When you notice your mind wandering, just focus on your breathing and bring your attention back to my voice.

(30 seconds)

Feel the sensation in your nose as the air touches it.

(15 seconds)

Become aware of the air as it fills your lungs till they are fully inflated.

(5 seconds)

Then, gently release your breath and feel as your lungs become deflated. Feel the air leave your body through the nose.

(5 Seconds)

Now, return to your normal breathing rhythm. Let your

breathing assume its own natural rhythm and just observe each inhale and exhale.

(30 seconds)

Remain alert and aware. If your mind wanders, bring your attention back to your breathing.

(30 seconds)

Now, notice the parts of your body that are in contact with the ground. Fell the support of the surface beneath you.

(10 seconds)

Direct your focus to your toes. Wiggle all your ten toes and feel them relaxing.

(10 seconds)

Make circles with your feet and let your ankles relax.

(10 seconds)

Notice your calf muscles and knees. Tighten the muscles around them and let go.

(10 seconds)

Bring your attention to your thighs, squeeze them together and release allowing them to relax.

(10 seconds)

Take your attention to your buttocks and feel them pressing down the surface beneath you. Relax them and let go of any tension around them.

(10 seconds)

Focus on your pelvic area and relax it.

(10 seconds)

Move your attention to your back. Do you feel any tension?

Tighten the muscles in your back and release them. Feel them relax as the tension around your back dissolves away.

(10 seconds)

Gently, take a deep breath through your nose and feel the air fill your entire body and then exhale completely releasing it.

(10 seconds)

Take a deep breath in and fill your belly completely allowing it to expand as much as possible and then exhale letting it fall and completely relax.

(10 seconds)

Round your shoulders and upper back and squeeze your chest muscles and then release and assume an upright position allowing the chest to open au.

(10 seconds)

Now, bring your attention to the shoulders. Squeeze them up towards your ears and then release them down letting go any tension as you feel them relax.

(10 seconds)

Stretch out your hands in front of you and make tight fists and then release spreading your fingers wide.

(10 seconds)

Rets your hands on your lap.

Drop your chin towards your collar bone and let the back of your neck stretch and release and tension.

(10 seconds)

Lift your chin as up as possible and allow the front of your neck to stretch and release tension.

(10 seconds)

Clench your jaw, close your eyes and tighten your facial muscles. Breath in deeply and hold your breath in for 7,6,5,4,3,2,1 and exhale gently as you allow your jaw and facial muscles to relax and then open your eyes.

(10 seconds)

Sit in the awareness of your entire body. It is relaxed and alert.

(30 seconds)

Bring back your attention to your breathing.

Inhale deeply and silently repeat the mantra 'I am inhaling.'

Exhale slowly as you silently say to yourself, 'I am exhaling.'

Keep breathing and reciting the mantras "I am inhaling", "I am exhaling".

(30 seconds)

When you notice your mind wandering, gently bring you attention back to your breathing and repeat the mantra.

I am inhaling.

I am exhaling

(30 seconds)

Gently direct your awareness to your body.

Feel the surface you are sitting on.

(5 seconds)

Notice the temperature on your skin.

(5 seconds)

Listen to the sounds around you.

(5 seconds)

Listen to your breathing.

(5 seconds)

Notice the sensations in your body.

(5 seconds)

Gently wiggle your fingers and your toes.

When you feel ready, open your eyes.

You are now ready to go on with your plans for the rest of the day.

Chapter 8
Guided Body Scan Meditation for Anxiety

Welcome to this body scan meditation. Think of the next 30 minutes as an opportunity to dwell in your body and to be in the present moment as it is.

(5 seconds)

Begin by finding a comfortable place to sit with your back straight but not stiff. If you are seated on a chair, allow your feet to rest on the ground. If you are seated on the ground, you may either cross your legs or straighten them. You could also do this meditation lying down with your feet extended in front of you and your hands resting beside your body. Adjust your body accordingly until you settle into a comfortable pose.

(10 seconds)

Gently close your eyes.

Become aware of the thoughts in your mind.

(10 seconds)

Our aim in this meditation is to release all the tension in your body and mind, so as to help you release stress and anxiety and to become calm and peaceful.

We will begin our scan from the top of our head to our toes. We will listen to our bodies and notice all the sensations then release all the tension and pains.

I will mention a part of your body; take your attention to that part of the body and scan it to detect any stress or tension around it. You will then visualize a yellow beam of energy shining on that part of the body as it washes away the pain, tightness or tension.

(5 seconds)

Now, bring your awareness to the top of your head and observe the sensations on this part of the body. Do you feel any tension? What sensations can you detect on this part of your body? Take a breath and send the energy light to it. See the light dissolve all the tension on the top of your head.

(20 seconds)

Bring your attention to your forehead. Is there tightness or any other noticeable sensation on this part of your body? Focus the yellow beam of energy to your forehead and let it melt away all the tension in this area.

(20 seconds)

Move your attention to your eyes. Scan them and check if they have any tension lodged in them. Do you feel any tightness behind your eyelids? Send the yellow beam of energy to the area around your eyes and feel as it dissolves the stress in your eyes.

(20 seconds)

Slowly move your awareness to your cheekbones and the cheeks. Observe whether there is any tension around them. Inhale and direct the yellow beam of energy on both cheeks allowing them to release tension and to relax.

(20 seconds)

Bring your awareness to your ears. Scan them for any tension and send the beam of energy to wash any tension that could be on your ears away.

(20 seconds)

Notice your mouth and jaw. Sense any tension around it. Shine the beam of energy on your mouth and jaw to clear away all that tension.

(20 seconds)

Become aware of your chin. Scan it for any tension. Now, shine the healing wave of energy to clear all the tension lodged in your chin. Feel as your chin relaxes.

(20 seconds)

Feel the back of your head. Slowly, scan it to detect any tension hidden in this area. Inhale deeply and let the yellow beam of energy consume all the tension held at the back of your head. As you exhale, allow your head to relax completely.

(20 seconds)

Take your awareness to your shoulders. Scan them for any tension. Now, send the energizing beam of energy to your shoulders and let it wash all the tension in that area.

(20 seconds)

Notice your chest. Notice how it rises and fall as you breathe in and out. Feel your heartbeat behind the chest. Scan every inch of your chest and check for tension lodged there. Focus the beam of energy to your chest. Let it clear all the tension, little by little until the entire chest area is fully relaxed.

(30 seconds)

Move your awareness to your back. Notice all the parts of your back from the upper back to the lower back, the spine and the entire torso. Scan the entire back for any tension, pain or tightness.

(5 seconds)

Shine the yellow beam of energy on your back. From the upper part of the back, to the middle part of the back and down to the lower back. Let this energizing light melt away any tension you are holding on to on your back.

(30 seconds)

Now, take your awareness to your stomach and the belly area. Visualize all the organs held within your rib cage and belly area. Your stomach, intestines, reproductive system, kidneys, liver, bladder, and all other organs. Scan your belly, ribcage and the organs beneath for tension or tightness.

(10 seconds)

Now, shine the beam of light to your stomach, rib cage and the organs beneath and let all the tension held on this area of the body dissolve.

(30 seconds)

Move your attention to your left arm.

Become aware of every part of your left arm; the biceps, triceps, forearm, palm and fingers.

(10 seconds)

Send the energy to your left arm to clear all the tension. Feel as the muscles in the whole of your left arm relax.

(10 seconds)

Now, move your awareness to your right arm. Notice all the parts of your right arm; biceps, triceps, forearm, palm and fingers. Scan for any tension in your arm.

(10 seconds)

Inhale and shine the beam of energy on your right arm and let all the tension in your right arm melt away. Feel as the right up relaxes.

(10 seconds)

Gently bring your awareness to your pelvis. Notice your buttocks, hips and groin area. Scan them for any tension, pain or tightness. Visualize the yellow beam of light shine upon your pelvis as it washes away all the tension leaving the buttocks, hips and groin completely relaxed.

(30 seconds)

Notice your left and right thighs. The thighs have the largest muscles in your body. As such, they can hold a lot of tightness and tension.

Bring your attention on the upper part of your right thigh and move your attention from the upper right thigh bit by bit up to the right knee as you scan for tension on the inner right thigh, top of the right thigh, back side of the right thigh and the outer edge of the right thigh. Now, visualize the relaxing beam of energy wash away tension from the upper part of the right thigh to knee.

(30 seconds)

Now, bring your attention on the upper part of your left thigh and move your attention from the upper left thigh bit by bit up to the left knee as you scan for tension on the inner left thigh, top of the left thigh, back side of the left thigh and the outer edge of the left thigh. Now, visualize the relaxing beam of energy wash away tension from the upper part of the left thigh to knee.

(30 seconds)

Become aware of the lower part of the legs. Notice your knees and the knee caps. Scan them for any tension and envision the yellow light dissolving all the tension that is on this part of your body.

(10 seconds)

Now, bring your attention to your left and right shins and calves.

(5 seconds)

Become aware of both of your ankles.

(5 seconds)

Scan your lower legs from the knees to your ankles for any pain or tension.

(10 seconds)

Inhale and shine the beam of energy beam on both of your legs from the knees to the ankles. As you exhale, feel your lower legs relax.

(15 seconds)

Gently move your awareness to your feet. Become aware of the bottom and the top part of your feet. Observe your feet and check for any tightness around them. Ease the tension there with the beam of light and feel as your feet relax.

(10 seconds)

Now envision the yellow beam of light shining on your entire body. It moves slowly from head to toes a sit washes away any remaining tension on your body.

(30 seconds)

It then moves from your toes to your head, bit by bit as it energizes every cell on your body.

(30 seconds)

Your body is now fully relaxed. You feel calm, peaceful, centered and grounded. Rest in this alert awareness of your body and in total relaxation for a moment.

(180 seconds)

Begin to deepen your breath. Gently wiggle your fingers and toes and when you are ready slowly open your eyes.

Chapter 9
Benefits of meditation

Meditation Helps to Reduce Stress

The modern-day lifestyle that we lead is hectic and inadvertently leads to stress and anxiety on some level. Stress has become one of the most common problems that people suffer from these days. You may think that you can put it off or might have resigned yourself to the fact that it is a part of your life. However, stress can lead to a myriad of health problems like high blood pressure, an increase in the risk of cardiovascular disorders, and insomnia, just to name a few. The stress chemical in the body is called cortisol. Your body can usually regulate the levels of cortisol within it, but the more your stress levels, the higher the amount of cortisol secreted. This can cause issues like panic attacks. Cortisol secretion needs to be regulated. All of these issues can, however, be dealt with using the help of meditation. It will help in reducing your stress levels and help you deal with anxiety-inducing issues in a productive manner. Overall, by practicing meditation, you will notice a decline in your stress and anxiety levels.

Meditation Helps Keep Emotions Under Control

Humans are emotional creatures. However, it can be hard for us to control our emotions at times, and this can have dangerous consequences. This is especially true in the present world that we live in. The increased amount of pressure and anxiety you experience can cause a build-up of many negative feelings. If you let emotions like anger build-up, it will only harm you. Not just you, but also those around you. Meditation will help you maintain your calm and stay composed even in the face of adversity. When you are able to stay calm, then it is easier to rationalize your thoughts. Apart from this, it will also help you make better decisions. You must not let your emotions control you, and meditation will help you get a handle on your emotions.

Meditation Increases Serotonin Secretion

You might have heard of serotonin, the "happy hormone." The human body secretes various hormones that have a huge impact on how you think and feel. These chemicals in your body will affect how happy, sad, or angry you are. Serotonin is a chemical that helps people stay happy. Studies show that regular meditation helps in increasing serotonin secretion. This chemical has a positive effect on your mind and body. Low levels of serotonin are observed in people suffering from depression and other mental health issues. So, meditation is one of the most effective means of tackling depression.

Meditation Improves the Ability to Focus

Having the ability to focus better is something everyone aims for in life. However, most people have trouble with this. Being able to focus can help you in so many ways. If you are a student, it will help you study better. If you have specific goals in life, you will be able to focus on those goals and work accordingly. Lack of focus can make you lose track of what you do and lead an undisciplined life.

Research shows that those who practice meditation tend to have a better ability to focus on their tasks and perform better than those who don't practice meditation. Different meditation techniques will help you hone your ability to focus and enhance your cognitive skills.

Meditation Increases Creativity

It is also said that meditation can get your creative juices flowing. When you meditate and reduce your stress levels, your brain is allowed to function better, and you can be more creative. This creative ability is often negatively impacted by high-stress levels. Meditation will help you embrace the good and the bad in your life without harming your happiness or health.

Meditation Increases Empathy and the Ability to Connect

You need to learn how to empathize and connect with others if you want better relationships. Meditation will help you learn compassion and thus act compassionately towards people. People who meditate tend to have an increased capacity for kindness and understanding towards others. You will be able to think of things from others' perspectives and react to situations in a better way. Meditation can enhance this empathetic ability and improve your social interactions.

Meditation Helps Improve Relationships

Do you feel like your relationships with your loved ones could use some extra help? Meditation can help you with this. Meditation helps increase your empathy, and this will help you immensely. It helps to increase your awareness so that you can pick up on cues from those around you. This will help you understand how they are feeling in certain situations. By getting a read on the situation, it will be easier for you to react and respond in the right way. Apart from this, it also helps reduce any chances of misunderstandings cropping up. Once your emotions are stabilized, the chances of letting any negativity through will decrease.

Meditation Enhances Memory

Do you feel like you have become forgetful? There could be many reasons behind this, stress being the main culprit. Regardless of what the cause is, meditation can help improve your memory, if practiced regularly. You will be able to focus on things and become more conscious of your surroundings and your own self. You will also be able to retain information for longer and thus be less forgetful. Meditation can be a great memory-enhancing tool regardless of what you do or what your age is.

Meditation Improves Immunity

Another benefit of meditation is that it is a holistic way of boosting your body's immune system. If you feel like you get sick too often or just want to be healthier, you should try meditation. Various meditation techniques like yoga are known to help in strengthening the immune system. By meditating regularly, you will notice a positive change in your overall immunity.

Meditation Helps You Overcome Addictions

Addictions are a serious affliction that can be really hard to contend with. It requires a lot of self-control and discipline to let go of any type of addiction. This could be smoking, alcoholism, or just about any unhealthy habit that has a negative impact on your health and well-being. It's not just the addictions that affect your physical health. There are other addictions like watching too much pornography, using excessive social media, binge eating, etc. These change your body and mind in many negative ways. There are certain meditation techniques, like Vipassana meditation, which is often used to help addicts overcome powerful addictions. Just meditating will not solve all your problems, but it is a great tool to help you move forward and leave your addictions behind. So, if you or anyone you know suffers from an addiction, trying meditation is a good place to start.

Meditation Benefits Cardiovascular Health

It is actually common sense that meditation is good for the heart. If you observe how regular meditation helps you when you need to relax and how it decreases your tendency to be anxious, at that point, is there any good reason why it shouldn't also help reduce the risk of cardiovascular issues, similar to hypertension?

For a considerable length of time, many assumed that to be the case, yet a couple of specialists appeared to be intrigued enough to research and document the physical outcomes on the heart after meditating. The leading researcher to explore this connection was Herbert Benson from Harvard. His important book, distributed in the mid-1970s, The Relaxation Response, raised a lot of discussions inside intellectual circles. Through medical testing, he showed that changes occurred in the body.

At first, other colleagues were skeptical of his discoveries. Nobody had ever genuinely thought that there could be medical advantages related to this meditative training. In any case, his testing withstood the thorough investigation conducted by others. In the last two decades, mainstream researchers picked up progressively genuine enthusiasm for the subject. The research started, yet more explicitly, the American Heart Association Journal published an article that reported the ability of meditation to bring down an individual's risk factors that are associated with all types of cardiovascular illness.

The American Journal of Hypertension recently also published positive on the medical advantages of meditation. In this research, it was found that a gathering of meditating people viably brought down their blood pressure, contrasted with a second group that didn't meditate. The decrease in blood pressure for these individuals was so apparent, truth be told, that the meditators had the option to reduce their utilization of antihypertensive drugs by about 25 percent. Stress is related to something beyond coronary illness.

Stress can cause disruption in a lot of physiological functions. At the end of the day, when you're worried all the time, it manifests in the form of any number of medical issues. One of the systems you may have noticed this in is through gastrointestinal dysfunctions. It's not "all in your head," it's been extensively recorded that changes in physiology and hormones happen in your body in relation to stress. These cause various stomach issues, as a response to a distressing condition - either acute or chronic.

A few people also experience sleep disorders due to stress. In some of these cases, sleep issues are linked with irritable bowel syndrome. Fortunately, these physical changes can be reduced and eased through consistent meditation practice.

Meditation Aids Weight Loss

It's hard to be your best when you're troubled with weight issues. Sadly, numerous people who are overweight do not have a good self-image and lack a sense of self-worth. Without that, they may believe that their ideal life is far out of their grasp. Meditation can do something amazing here, in two different ways. To begin with, it's not unusual to start eating when you're stressed out.

If you are someone who does this, you realize that what you go after first is generally something salty, sugary or greasy. It's not about your absence of self-restraint - blame the hormonal changes related to too much stress instead. Your body craves this kind of unhealthy food when it is under distress.

A lot of research demonstrates that the physical impact of stress on your body can be greatly diminished through meditation. It starts by diminishing the body's cortisol level, which can then mitigate those obstinate yearnings for food. Maybe meditating doesn't offer that equivalent comfort that you get from the bag of chips, candy, or fries (or even all three). Yet, it can help curb those cravings in any case. This is a part of the process that will allow people to pick up a superior mental self-image, which, then, empowers them to concentrate on seeking the life that they need to lead. Stress is very slippery. It penetrates your entire being. Maybe, however, its most notable impending impacts are on the person's immunity. Consider it. How often have you caught a cold or even the flu following an unpleasant event?

Meditation can definitely help you with this also. People under pressure are known to have decreased amounts of basic white blood cells, which are essential for battling foreign attacking microscopic organisms and infections, which can cause cold, influenza, and other illnesses. Meditation is undoubtedly now seen as a great way to insightfully deal with the stress in your life.

Meditation Helps Manage Headaches

A headache is one of the most common signs that your body is experiencing too much stress. What's more, it's difficult to concentrate on what is important to you when a headache is floating over the majority of your thoughts. It's hard to think, and at the same time, it's hard to use sound judgment, and it's tough to enjoy yourself. Maybe it doesn't come as anything unexpected that meditation is the ideal method to loosen up those muscles and suppress that pain.

In addition to the fact that it works for most people, its positive effects are likewise scientifically confirmed. Even for a brief timeframe, going within yourself as meditation allows you to make changes in your brain waves to another higher state. This is a dimension of awareness that is known to help advance the process of healing. The takeaway here is that through meditation, you can adjust your brain waves. Researchers were once convinced that an individual's brain waves are unchangeable. They trusted that we are brought into the world with specific patterns, and these couldn't be modified, despite our ability to switch between different dimensions of cognizance.

Today, however, it's broadly acknowledged that your brain waves can be changed—and meditation is one way in which this can be accomplished. The most recent studies have taken a look at people who have been meditating for over fifteen years. Long-term meditation changes the functioning of the brain, which permits the individuals who meditate to achieve a more elevated amount of mindfulness than the individuals who don't. In any case, nothing is preventing you right now from disposing of that migraine through a ten-or fifteen-minute session of meditation, so why not try it?

As you can see, meditation has a lot of benefits for those who practice it regularly. There are actually more ways in which it helps than just the ones mentioned above. If you genuinely want to experience the benefits of meditation, you need to get started.

How Can I Establish A Good Meditation Practice?

One effective way to consistently practice meditation is to create and plan out a practice that you can follow, according to your needs, your daily schedule, routines, and timing.

The thing about meditation is that you need to be mindful of everything that you experience in your session. With mindful meditation, there is a goal and a purpose. It is to help you be conscious and mindful of everything you do.

Benefits Of Establishing A Meditation Practice

A foundation of your meditation session is important because, in many ways, when you set the stones to your practice, your brain will start moving toward making this practice happen. For example, if you decide to buy a new meditation mat, your mind will be reminded (or you will remember) that you purchased the mat, and you want to know the feeling of sitting on the mat and practicing.

Without a firm foundation, you will not be consistent

It won't be long before whatever you're doing eventually crumbles and falls because there's nothing supporting it. That's just one way of describing how important it is to develop a sound meditation practice right from the very beginning of the process.

It helps you create a habit

But although meditation is something that is beneficial for everyone, not everyone is currently putting it into practice. Some people are not practicing meditation at all. Why? Because it isn't a habit. A lot of us lead very busy lives, so sometimes our plates seem too full to take on anything else. There will always be a reason not to start something, which is why it is entirely up to you to make time for it.

The purpose of establishing a meditation practice is because you want to make meditation a habit, a part of your daily life, and something that you are willing to do every day without even thinking twice or resisting it because you are pressed for time.

It makes your practice ingrained, almost second-nature activity in your life

Meditating will become much like how brushing your teeth or showering, preparing something to eat, and even going on a daily commute to work. Those habits are so deeply ingrained in you that you do them without any effort or a lot of thought put into it.

That is what establishing a meditation practice aims to do for you right now, and it is something you need to establish as a foundation to make your practice consistent

Chapter 10
Mindfulness Meditation

When we experience stress and anxiety, it is often simply worrying over the past or fears that we are having about the future. The best way to overcome these constant fears is to be mindful in the present moment to keep your thoughts grounded in reality. In this meditation, we are going to help you stay mindful so that you can focus on what matters the most—healing.

You cannot heal if your thoughts and emotions are glued to some time period that is out of your control. You cannot change the past, so guilt and remorse are only going to keep you stuck in a different dimension. No matter how prepared we can be for the future, there is still a level of unpredictability that we will never be able to conquer. In this meditation, you are going to learn exactly what it means to stay in the present moment to start the healing process.

Meditation for Self-Healing Mindfulness

For this meditation, you will want to be in a completely comfortable place. It is preferred that you do this meditation when you are able to fall asleep afterwards, but that's also not entirely necessary. Doing this outside where you can take a nap with nature would also be an excellent way to fully feel the beneficial effects of this meditation.

This is going to be a visualization exercise that will help take your mind to a calm and relaxed place. You will remove any thoughts that are keeping you glued to some time period which you cannot change. In order to really feel the benefit of this meditation, focus on your breathing and keep a clear mind.

Anytime that a thought starts to travel into your mind, gently push it away. You do not have to force them out of your mind. You do not have to block out negative thoughts and punish yourself for having them. Simply let them drift in and out like a car passing you by. There is no need to latch onto these thoughts and you don't need to shove them to a corner of your brain. Let them come into your mind and push them out as soon as they do.

Focus on your breathing once again. Breathe in through your nose for five and out through your mouth for five. Breathe in for one, two, three, four, and five, and out for five, four, three, two, and one.

Keep every part of your body relaxed and let your eyes gently close. No need to hold them closed tightly to the point that you are straining yourself. Let your eyelids gently stay shut. We are going to count down from twenty. When we reach one, you will be into the meditation. Let your mind become completely black and continue to feel the air come in and out of your body.

Breathe in for five and out for five.

Your mind is completely blank. You do not see anything at all. The only thing your mind is focused on now is feeling the air continue to cycle throughout your body.

In your mind, you start to see a small bright dot. The dot continues to grow bigger and bigger until you discover that you are engulfed in sunlight.

You look around and discover that you are surrounded by lush, green trees. Each thing that you see around you is a reminder that you are a part of nature. All of these various aspects are part of a living ecosystem in which you are also operating at this moment. Breathe in the fresh air and feel as it fills your body.

As you look in front of you, you see that there is a little trail between some of the trees. You take a step forward and begin to walk around. You can feel as the dirt and the leaves crunch beneath your feet. It is a beautiful fall day, and the orange and yellow changing of the trees is filling you with a sense of warmth. There's a light breeze but nothing that is keeping you too chilled in this moment. You can see bits of the sky above you. Bright blue is beaming through the break of the leaves. You continue to walk forward and see in front of you that there is a very large path. Now, many individuals have already walked down this path themselves before. You are not concerned with what has happened over the past or the potentials of the future. You are completely grounded in the present moment, and only focused on this at the time being. Breathe in this good energy and breathe out anything that has been keeping you trapped in a place which you do not have control. Everything that you have experienced leading up to this moment has brought you to be the exact person that you are. Even if you are not happy with who this person is at the present moment, there will be one day where everything makes sense. You will be able to look back on your past and know that each struggle was just another step towards making you the individual that you are. Not everything has been easy for you up until this point, but it has been a learning experience that teaches you something greater about yourself. Breathe in now as you begin to accept the things that have happened in your past. Breathe out as you are letting go of any of the emotions that you have experienced. You continue to walk towards more and more trees, and you think about how nature is so incredible. You are a part of all of these living things. No matter what these trees and flowers and other little plants might experience, they continue to live on. There is nobody tending to them.

These plants don't have a gardener who comes and makes sure that they are free from any diseases or root rot. Nobody is watering them and nurturing them. They're able to take care of themselves on their own because they are a part of a larger system. Bugs help to keep them pollinated and plants around them will also aid in the way that they grow. Animals might come and feast on them, and they soak up as much sun and rain as they possibly can.

This is a reminder of the powerful ability that all living things have to carry on, no matter what the circumstances might be. Your body will always be there and provide you with the nourishment and fulfillment that is needed to make sure that you are as healthy as possible. No matter what you give to your body, whether it is something healthy, or a type of junk food, you will be able to take the most important and beneficial aspects of this using your body. Everything that exists inside of you is something that happens on its own. You don't have to tell your body how to process and break down food. It naturally does this all. All of this is a reminder that you are a part of a greater living organism. This earth is flowing around so freely and gently, as it should be. You continue to walk forward, and you notice that there is a little pond. You walk up to it and see that there are some little fish swimming around in the bottom. These fish could be a source of food.

These fish could be somebody else's family. These fish are their own living organisms, and they are simply existing. They swim against the current, and they look for food on the top of the surface. No matter what they might experience, their main focus will always be on continuing to live. It is a powerful reminder that when you feel lost, you can always rest assured that your intention and purpose is to simply carry on living, breathing.

Breathe in as you notice the site and breathe out as you let go of any sort of thoughts that are keeping you glued somewhere else. It is okay to think and plan for the future. And we all have moments where we reflect on the past. The issue comes when you obsess over these things. If you are only thinking in different time periods, other than what is occurring now, then you will not be able to give your full energy to the things that are currently surrounding you. Breathe in the excitement over staying mindful and productive in this moment. Breathe out any desire to stay stuck in a different time period.

You look down and notice the fish. You could grab any one of them that you wanted. This pond isn't that large and not that deep. You would probably be able to pick one up as long as you gave it a few tries.

This is something within your power, and you have a choice. You choose not to and instead let these fish continue swimming on. There's no point in taking one of these fish from the pond. Sure, you might be able to use it for food later, but you don't need that. You simply continue to watch as these fish float around. You don't scare them away and you don't try to move them. They're simply there. This is how we need to start to treat our thoughts. Our thoughts can sometimes just be like fish swimming around in a fishbowl. The thoughts will always be there. They won't go away. The thing is, you don't have to feed these fish. You don't have to pick them up. You don't have to move them around. You don't have to kill them. You don't have to do anything. You can simply let them continue to swim around and around. Your thoughts do not have to be given attention. These thoughts can come into your mind, but you don't have to be afraid and push them out so negatively. Instead, you can simply focus on yourself and create a positive and healthy mindset. When you have negative thoughts, remember that they can simply swim away like fish. Breathe in and out, in and out.

You sit next to the pond and close your eyes once again. You dip your toes down into the cool water. Even though it is a fall day, it is not freezing just yet and instead the water gives you a reminder of the last little bit of summer that's left. Breathe in and out, in and out. You close your eyes and lay back against a thick layer of leaves on the ground. You feel completely comfortable, at peace and at ease. Breathe in and out, in and out.

You close your eyes, and everything starts to fade away once again. All is becoming black and there are no thoughts left that are travelling through your mind.

This is a safe and relaxing place that you can travel back to anytime that it is needed. You are completely at ease and peace is seeping out of every last one of your pores. You have no thoughts that are keeping you stuck in a negative place now. You cannot heal unless you are relaxed and free from the fears that have been holding you back for so long. Breathe in for one, two, three, four, and five, and out for five, four, three, two, and one.

Continue to feel yourself relax. You are sinking deeper and deeper and further and further into the couch. There isn't a single thing that is keeping you held back in this moment. You are entirely relaxed and at ease. We are going to count down from twenty once again.

Chapter 11
How to meditate

Meditation is a great - and logically demonstrated - habit for a solid body and mind. Be that as it may, a few people battle with the time, consistency, center, and system required to get meditation right.

What great many people don't know is, you don't really need to take a seat and close your eyes for a considerable length of time a day - in light of the fact that there are other far less demanding approaches to get your psyche into a thoughtful state, and appreciate the advantages of this ancient practice.

For example:

1. While you walk your dog

As you're strolling Jack, instead of meditating a large number of things you're stalling on, take a stab at giving careful attention to your environment.

Recognize the sounds, the general population, the climate. What do you smell? What would you be able to see? What would you be able to hear out yonder? How does your body feel?

By taking a careful walk, you're discharging endorphins, which enable you to build your joy level, and even diminish stress and live longer.

2. *While you make coffee or tea*

- Begin your morning with more profound concentration, lucidity, and peace by rehearsing this simple reflective custom.

- As you make your tea or coffee, concentrate your attention on your developments.

- Close your eyes and notice the tea, take a taste, enjoy it. Furthermore, as you experience the ritual custom, be deliberately mindful of your breath.

- You can likewise apply this while you cook your most loved supper or heat.

3. *While you do the dishes*

- Doing dishes or clearing your floor doesn't need to be an errand. Actually, this is the ideal time for you to associate with yourself and feel grounded.

- Concentrate on your breath and your body's sensations.

- On the off chance that you see your mind wandering, take yourself back to mindfulness by thinking about the general population and things throughout your life that fill you with delight and appreciation.

4. *While you shower*

- Have you at any point asked why your best thoughts tend to come while you're showering?

- "The shower is where we can develop mindfulness. When we get tranquil, when we get still, when we rest, you could state, in mindfulness, our natural drive to see associations that we didn't see the prior minute is unobstructed."

- On the off chance that you need to take it somewhat further, as you shower, you can even envision accomplishing your objectives and the feeling that will wash over you as you do.

5. While you tune in to your main tune

- Practicing mindfulness or meditation can be as straightforward as tuning in to your main song - insofar as you're totally centered around your breathing and the feeling that the song brings out in you.

6. While you ride the transport or sit in your auto

- Sit serenely. Take long and full breaths. Recognize the warm sun stroking your face. Welcome the delightful city lights or scenes. Also, let your mind take you all alone trip.

As you now know, the benefits of meditation can be conveyed into the most ordinary exercises - helping you acknowledge life all the more, inhabit a slower pace, embrace new propensities, and be more joyful.

Practical Advice on meditation

To what extent Should I Meditate?

In the event that you are new to meditation, I suggest

beginning gradually. Begin with only 5 minutes every day. Bit by bit increment the time more than half a month. When I began reflecting, five minutes felt like an unfathomable length of time. I now practice for 30 minutes every day, and here and there, I am astonished at how rapidly it passes!

Where Should I Meditate?

Locate a comfortable spot where you can sit. You can sit on the floor (utilizing a pad or pad for help if necessary) or sit upright in a seat, with your feet laying on the floor.

A few people suggest that you shouldn't rest on your back; however, I figure you ought to think in whatever stance works for you (unless resting influences you to fall asleep!)

You can meditate anyplace, yet I like having an extraordinary place in my home for my training. You can take in more about making a meditation space in your home here.

What Do I Do?

The least demanding meditation strategy is to count the breath. I forget about each in-breath and breath with a similar number. So my mind concentrates on "One" (in-breath), "One" (out-breath), "Two" (in-breath), "Two" (out-breath), et cetera. When I hit 10 (which seldom occurs before my mind has wandered!), I begin once again at one. On the off chance that you don't care for counting, you can essentially rehash to yourself "in, out... . in, out... "

At the point when your mind wanders, which it WILL DO (that's what the mind does!) tenderly guide your attention back to your breath. On the off chance that you have to begin once again counting in light of the fact that you don't recollect the latest relevant point of interest, that is fine! The key is to not reprimand or judge yourself for giving your attention a chance to wander. Actually … seeing that your psyche has wandered is the general purpose of meditation, you are winding up more mindful of the activities of your mind!

Indeed, even the moderately basic guideline to "take after the breath" can sound somewhat obscure or confounding. A supportive method is to bring your attention where you most notice the vibe of the breath — in the chest and lungs? the nose? the stomach? That is your stay. Each time your mind wanders, return to the physical vibes of relaxing.

At the point when thought emerges, it's anything but difficult to get diverted and tail them and draw in them and explain them and investigate them… . An accommodating practice is just to name the contemplations: "stressing," "arranging," "recollecting." Don't stress over making sense of the exact mark for the kind of thought you're having. Simply "considering" will do, as well!

What's more, if the thoughts don't leave? It's still alright.

I adore that depiction of the training.

How Do I Fit This Into My Day?

The critical thing is to make it a propensity. After numerous long stretches of a reliable practice, it will end up being a vital piece of your day, such as practicing or brushing your teeth!

Changing your habits over some stretch of time really makes new neural systems in your mind, and the training will turn out to be a piece of your day by day schedule.

Knocks along the Road.

In any case, Nothing's Happening!

Meditation is about non-judgmental mindfulness. We have not to bring desires into our practice. You may encounter a snapshot of significant understanding amid a meditation session. Or, then again, you may be truly exhausted. You may feel fretful and disturbed. Or, on the other hand, you may feel quiet and relaxed.

Meditation is tied in with grasping whatever is right now. The advantages of meditation — more noteworthy mindfulness and discretion, increased calm and empathy — will rise after some time. In any case, every individual session will be totally unique.

So, in case you're exhausted, simply take note of, "This is the thing that fatigue feels like." If you're content, take note of, "This is the thing that satisfaction feels like."

- Meditating for 10 minutes daily is limitlessly superior to meditating for 70 minutes once per week. Attempt to meditate oftentimes (consistently if conceivable), regardless of the possibility that that just means sitting for a couple of minutes.

- Start little. In the event that you endeavor to meditate for 30 minutes right from the beginning, I can practically ensure that you will get disappointed and disheartened. I prescribe beginning with five minutes, and just increase that time when you're comfortable. Regardless of the possibility that you sit for five minutes, and you find that your mind wanders the entire time, you will, in any case, get unfathomable advantages from meditation.

- Pick a gentle alarm. On the off chance that your clock is uproarious and jolting, reckoning the caution will occupy your attention amid meditation.

- Meditate in a peaceful place. Having fewer distractions around you will normally enable you to meditate better, and will make your meditation significantly more profitable.

- It's most straightforward to lose your attention amid your out-breath. Your in-breath is exceptionally articulated and simple to focus on, and the vast majority's mind wanders on their out-breaths (me included). These merits remembering.

- Be simple on yourself when your mind wanders. It's anything but difficult to wind up plainly disappointed with yourself when your mind wanders, yet don't. Your meditations will be substantially more gainful when you delicately bring your mind back.

Chapter 12
How to Practice Mindfulness Meditation

Unlike other types of meditation, being mindful doesn't require a large time commitment or a space that is quiet and calm for a specific period of time. While these things will certainly help you get into the required mindset at first, eventually, you will find that you can get your mindfulness on while at the gym, doing chores, or even commuting to and from work. Regardless of where you do it, the basics of mindfulness meditation are always the same.

Stick with a specific time

As with any new habit, it is crucial that you create a routine around your mindfulness meditation practices for the best results. Generally speaking, you can expect it to take about 30 days for a new habit to really stick, which means that you will need to commit to going hard for just four weeks before you can expect to start seeing the best results.

Unfortunately, due to its few requirements and low impact nature, it is often quite easy to push off your set mindfulness meditation time for a later than never comes, especially if they are already very busy as it stands. If you find yourself always coming up with an excuse to get out of meditating at the moment, you may find the following piece of advice particularly useful. "Practice mindfulness meditation for fifteen minutes every day unless, of course, you are extremely busy, in which case you should practice for thirty minutes instead." Don't let the outside world intrude on your potential for inner peace, find a time each day that works for you and stick with it no matter what; in a month's time, you will be glad you did.

Find a quiet place

In order to reach a state of mindfulness, you are going to want to find someplace comfortable, and quiet to sit, though not so quiet and comfortable that you are tempted to fall asleep. Then, all you need to do is breathe deeply, in and out.

Breathe

Start by doing your best to calm your mind by taking a few deep breaths and then announce your intentions aloud to make them more tangible. From there, take several more deep breaths and focus on the sensations that your senses are providing you as you do so. Consider how your lungs feel as they expand and the smells this action brings to your attention. If you are sitting, consider the feel of the chair on your skin, the temperature of the room, and the movement of any wind across your skin. Let the sensations flow from one to another, working their way down your body completely.

Continue breathing deeply, but keep your eyes and ears alert and providing you with more information than you previously thought possible. Focus on this information to the exclusion of everything else. You will likely find it difficult to shut out the constant flow of information that is running through your mind relating to things you need to do, regrets over past actions and plans that must be made, but this is completely normal. If you find your focus drifting away from the moment, take note of the mistake and move on. There is nothing to be gained from beating yourself up over it, and you will only take yourself out of the moment even more.

Visualize

Once you have reached a relaxed state, to remove the excess thoughts that are likely running through your head, all you need to do is picture them as a stream of bubbles that are rushing by in front of your eyes. Simply take a step back and let the thoughts flow past you without interacting with them. If one of them catches your attention and draws you into more complex thought, simply disengage and let it go. Don't focus on the fact that you were thinking about it, because that will just draw you out of the moment, simply remain in that state for as long as possible. Eventually, this will help with negative thoughts you experience in the real world as well.

In fact, with enough time and practice, you will likely find that you are able to maintain a mild meditative state even when you are otherwise focused on the world around you. This is known as a state of mindfulness, and it should be the end goal of everyone who is new to the meditative practice. Being mindful means always being connected to a calming and soothing mental state as well as one that is full of joy and peace, which benefits not just yourself but everyone around you.

Ignore those pesky judgments

Mindfulness is not necessarily quieting the mind or finding an eternal state of calmness. The goal here is simple. You want to pay attention to the moment you are in without judging it. When you judge a thought or something you may have done in the past, you likely, tend to dwell on it. That isn't living in the moment and is not conducive to mindful meditation. While this is easier said than done, it is a crucial step to mindful meditation. With practice, it will be easy to achieve. Be mindful of the moment, of your senses and your surroundings.

Take notice of the times you are passing judgment while practicing mindfulness. Make a note of them and move on. It is easy for your mind to get lost in thought. Mindfulness meditation is the art of bringing yourself back to the moment, over and over, as many times as it takes. Don't get discouraged. In the beginning, you will find your mind wanders a lot. Reel it back in and keep moving forward. Even if your mind does happen to wander, and it will, don't be hard on yourself. It happens. Acknowledge whatever thoughts pop up, put them to the side, and get back on track.

Keep it up

When you first start practicing mindfulness meditation, it is very important that you do so under the understanding that you aren't going to see any results from your hard work at first and rather need to commit to the process fully before you can start receiving any rewards. Specifically, you will need to keep in mind that it is natural for your mind to wander freely for a time before you are able to guide it to where it needs to be. To better understand the mindset that you should be striving for, you might find it useful to consider the moment of complete blankness the mind experiences once it has heard a question, but before it can generate an answer.

Tips For Meditation

We will share some more suggestions and tips to allow you to continue with your meditation practice. These are not aimed at making you an expert but just to assist you on the journey. It is not necessary to try all of these tips at the same time. You can try one or two at a time to see if they help you. There will be some that work better than others. Find what's right for you.

Begin Your Practice with 2-Minute Sessions

It may sound like it's pointless to meditate for just two minutes, but trust us when we say it's anything but. It's simple to do this and is the easiest way for a beginner to learn to practice meditation. Just dedicate two minutes of each day to meditation. Continue this for a week. It's easier to follow through with these two minutes than pressuring yourself to sit still for half an hour. Once you get used to these two minutes, you can add more minutes the next week and so on. You will soon see that you easily meditate at least 15 minutes daily after a couple of weeks, and that will be more than enough time for most. So don't worry and don't make excuses about not having time. Everyone has two minutes to meditate.

Practice Your Meditation Every Morning

A lot of people say that they will meditate every day in the beginning, but most of them fail to follow through with this claim. Don't assume that you will always remember or be inclined to do it. Commit yourself to meditate every single morning after you wake up. After you wash up, just set aside a few minutes for this, and you will see how much better your day goes. Early mornings are considered the best time to meditate.

Don't Worry About the Process and Focus on Beginning the Practice

When people start meditating or think about starting it, they often waste a lot of time and energy on worrying about how they should go about it. They waste time in looking up too many methods, finding the perfect mat to sit on, learning chants, etc. All of these are a part of the practice but not the essence of it. You need not spend so much time on this and should try to go with the flow. Just find a comfortable place to sit where you won't be disturbed or distracted by anything. Sitting right on the ground is completely fine, and so is sitting on a chair. To begin with, focus less on all this and more on spending two whole minutes just meditating. The stress of these trivial things will hinder your meditation. So try to get more used to meditating itself and worry about all this later.

Pay Attention to How You Feel

Once you begin meditating, you need to try being more attuned to your personal feelings. Pay attention to how you feel and how this practice is affecting your body. Tune in to the thoughts that pass through your mind. Don't focus on them but notice them as they flow past. Be accepting of all the feelings and thoughts that you experience during meditation. Nothing is wrong or right, so don't judge yourself for any of it.

Count as You Breathe

Breathing is an important aspect of meditation. Find the right place to meditate and then close your eyes as you sit comfortably. Start concentrating solely on your breathing. Focus on your breath as you inhale and exhale. Notice how you take in air through your nose and into your lungs. Pay attention as it leaves your body. When you take in a breath, count one. Count two when you breathe out. Continue the counting as you keep breathing and focus on this alone. It will help you focus more.

It Is Okay for Your Thoughts to Wander

The human mind tends to wander a lot, and you need to be more accepting of it as you meditate. You don't have to assume that you are not allowed to think anything when you meditate. This can be impossible to avoid, at least at first. When you meditate, try not to think but be accepting when thoughts come in. When you notice your concentrating wandering off from your meditation to your thoughts, push back your mind slowly. It can be disappointing, and you might feel like you are doing it wrong, but it is all right. Just slowly come back when your mind wanders away.

Be More Accepting

Like we already said, it is natural for thoughts to appear as you meditate. Don't be defensive, and try to push them away all the time. Instead, be more accepting and allow them to come and pass. Take note of these thoughts, and you can focus on them later. But as you meditate, allow them to come and go naturally. Your thoughts are a part of you, and you need to accept and forgive yourself for everything that you are.

Don't Stress About the Method of Meditation

You might be worried that you are meditating the wrong way at first. A lot of people get stressed about this and think it will be ineffective if they don't practice the right method or do it the right way. The truth is, there is no perfect method of meditation. You can try the various methods we have mentioned and use them as guidelines, but ultimately, you need to do what feels best for you.

Your Mind Doesn't Have to be Empty While Meditating

Some people think that meditation means getting rid of all thoughts and clearing the mind completely. However, this is not true and can be almost impossible for most people. It can be possible to clear your mind out sometimes, but for the most part, it's not what is essential for meditation. It's normal to have thoughts, and you don't have to force yourself to push them all out. Just be more accepting of them and let them pass without focusing on them. Work more on your concentration, and you will see that it gets easier to reduce distracting thoughts over time.

Take Some Time to Accept Your Thoughts and Feelings

Having thoughts while meditating is totally normal. When a thought passes through your mind, it is okay to take a moment and pay attention to it. In the beginning, we recommend to just let the thoughts pass and focus more on breathing. But over time, you can try noticing more of your thoughts too. You should avoid focusing on anything negative and try to bring in more positive thoughts. When you notice your thoughts, you will be able to learn more about yourself. But only allow yourself a moment for this before continuing with your meditation.

Learn a Little More About Yourself Every Day

Meditation is not just about improving your focus or being better able to concentrate. It is about helping your mind develop too. When you become more accepting of your thoughts and feelings, you will learn a lot about yourself. Don't push yourself too hard to think or feel a certain way. Be accepting and learn about yourself. No one can know you better than yourself.

Be Your Own Friend

You need to try learning more about yourself, but this should not be done with a mindset of self-analysis and judgment. Instead, be kinder to yourself. Think of it like learning more about someone you like. Accept who you are and be your friend. Don't be cruel and judgmental towards yourself.

Pay Attention to Your Body

After you get better at counting breaths and meditating, you can try something else. Now you should try focusing on your body. Do this with one body part at a time. As you meditate, focus on a specific body part and try to pay attention to how it feels. Start with the lowest point in your body and move on until every part of your body has been acknowledged. This will allow you to pay attention to your body and learn more about it. You will be able to notice if something feels wrong too.

Be Truly Determined

You cannot say you will meditate regularly and then fail to follow through. It is important to dedicate yourself to this practice. Don't take it lightly. Make sure you stick to this resolution for at least a few weeks. Motivate yourself to follow through with it every day. It will soon become a habit, but not if you lack determination right from the beginning.

Meditate, Regardless of Where You Are

It doesn't matter if you're on a trip or have to work overtime on some days. Don't skip your meditation practice. You might reduce the amount of time you can dedicate to it, but you should still meditate. You don't necessarily need that meditation corner in your home for this. It can be done while sitting in a car or even while you sit in your office chair.

Use Guided Meditations

It may seem hard to meditate when you first begin. Guided meditations can be instrumental in this case. Use these audio or video files to help you get started. They are very simple and accommodating regardless of whether you are a beginner or have practiced for some time.

Have Someone to Be Accountable To

If you keep by yourself your resolution to meditate, you are less likely to follow through with it. It will be easy to give up because there is no one to berate you over it. This is why you need to have someone that will hold you accountable. It could be a friend or family member. Just keep checking in with them, and they will help you stay on track. You can also find someone to practice it regularly. This could be someone you live with, work with, or even someone who will go to lessons with you. Finding a network of people who are interested in meditation will help in reinforcing your new good habit. These people can help support you through your journey. You can find online forums or communities of people who practice meditation too.

Chapter 13
Dealing with Stress

Stress, however unpleasant, is a normal reaction that occurs in our body and is sometimes beneficial. It is the body's response to changes that are occurring and require adjustment or response. These responses can be physical, mental, or emotional. As a normal part of life, stress can be triggered by everyday things around us such as our environment, our thoughts, and our body. These stressors can either be positive such as getting married or negative such as getting fired from job. The more stressors you experience, the more load you are likely to feel on your nervous system. Simply put, stress can be defined as the feeling we get when we're overwhelmed and struggling to cope with demands. Even so, anything that poses a threat or challenge, real or perceived, causes stress.

Stress acts as an indicator of danger and is thus beneficial for our survival. This is where the 'fight or flight' response comes to play. Stress flushes our body systems with hormones to help us confront or evade danger by telling us when and how to react to danger. This is the fight or flight mechanism and is the reason stress can be defined as the body's natural defense against danger. This mechanism always fuels a physical reaction –that is to either get away from the situation or stay and fight the stressor. Following the flush of hormones, our bodies tend to produce larger quantities of chemicals and hormones such as adrenaline, cortisol, and noradrenaline that in turn cause a specific

GUIDED MEDITATIONS FOR ANXIETY

response in the body such as increased heart rate, alertness, sweating and muscle preparedness all which will aid the final response of fight or flight.

Stress is helpful and can be a motivator; in this context it is referred to as eustress –that is positive stress that keeps us productive and on the go. In many cases, it helps save our lives by helping us react in a way to stop or prevent danger, for example, jerking off the road when you see a car coming your way. In other cases, it serves as a motivator, for instance, helping you focus on a project that's due or keeping you on guard during a presentation or speech. We all experience and go through stress differently but like everything else, too much of it is dangerous and can lead to health problems.

Effects of Chronic Stress

Our nervous systems are not good at distinguishing between physical and emotional threats. For instance, your body cannot distinguish between the stressed caused by an exam or a robber in front of you. In either case, your body is likely to give off the same reaction. The more your stress systems are activated the easier you can be triggered and the harder it is to get out of a state of constant stress. This is referred to as chronic stress and is the most harmful form of stress- it goes on for long periods and occurs when one never sees the end to a stressor and stops finding solutions.

This is even more common in today's demanding society. This leads us to get used to it and become unnoticeable as it makes up part of our personalities. Nowadays, our bodies are in a constant heightened state of stress, which more often than not leads to serious health problems. Stress disrupts almost all of one's body systems and can rewire the brain causing one to be vulnerable to anxiety, depression, other mental illnesses and in other cases, it can cause heart attacks, strokes, violent actions, and suicide.

While stress is usually a short-term experience of your body's reaction to a trigger, anxiety is a sustained mental disorder that is triggered by prolonged periods of stress. Anxiety does not usually fade away once the stressor is evaded, on the contrary, it stays for long and can cause impairment and damage to areas of functioning such as societal involvement and one's occupational responsibilities.

Signs and Symptoms of Chronic Stress

It is important to understand and be aware of the common signs of stress overload as you may get used to indulging in stressful situations and not pay much attention to the damage it's causing to your health and wellbeing.

Emotional Signs and Symptoms

Feeling overwhelmed
Agitation and anxiety
Anger, mood swings and feeling irritable
Isolation and loneliness
Irritability
Forgetfulness
Anger
Restlessness
Insecurity
Fatigue

Sadness and depression

Rise of mental or emotional health problems

Cognitive Signs and Symptoms

Racing thoughts

Poor judgment

Memory problems

Anxious thoughts

Constant worrying

Pessimism and negativity

Concentration problems

Behavioral Signs and Symptoms

Insomnia

Oversleeping

Relationship problems

Frequent crying

Eating more or less than usual

Cravings

Sudden anger outbursts

Substance abuse to relax

Procrastination and laziness

Neglecting responsibilities

Nervous habits such as shaking one's leg or nail-biting

Withdrawal from society

Physical Signs and Symptoms

Nausea or dizziness

Loss of sex drive

Increased heart rate

Chest pains

Aches and pains

Nervous twitches

Stomach upset

Various diseases

Fainting

Frequent flu and/or colds

Constipation or Diarrhea

Anger Management

Anger describes an unpleasant emotion characterized by strong feelings of antagonism and displeasure that ranges from mild irritability or annoyance to intense fury or rage. Our triggers for anger differ from person to person, however, we are exposed to these triggers often. Anger is a normal human emotion that when recognized and appropriate action is taken to deal with it can bear positive outcomes. In this case, it may even become a motivator inspiring one to advocate for social change or stand up for certain injustices. Anger notifies us when we need to take action and rectify something while giving us the motivation, strength, and energy to act. However, when anger is unresolved or left unchecked it can lead to inappropriate and/or aggressive behavior. In this case, it may be referred to as a 'negative' emotion.

Over the past few years especially in the industrial and the now post-industrial era, there has been a significant and continuous rise in stress and anger. This shows that stress has a role in influencing anger. If one is more prone to anger then a lot of stress is likely to trigger feelings of anger. When stress becomes too much and ceases to be a motivator, it may cause us to feel irritable or just angry to the core. When this happens, one is usually overwhelmed with tons of stressors and typically one feels like they lack the resources to deal with stress effectively and has an outburst of anger. This type of stress is referred to as distress. If stressors are understood and steps are taken to maintain equilibrium and deal with the stress, then one can limit distress thereby controlling and limiting one's anger.

Techniques for Anger Relaxation and Management

Techniques for anger relaxation are frequently used in anger management therapy to help us understand our anger and act in ways that are positive to alleviate the negative aspects of anger rather than suppress feelings of anger. These techniques work most effectively when practiced frequently. Some of the techniques are as follows:

Controlled Deep Breathing

When we get angry, several subtle physical changes occur and notify us of these feelings. One of the most noticeable is the change in breathing. When one is angry or upset, their breathing becomes shallow and quick. Noticing this is one of the first steps of this technique. Once one noticed the change in breath, one can make a deliberate effort to deepen and slow their breathing –this will help in maintaining control. These breaths ought to come from your belly rather than your chest. The breaths should be twice as long when coming out as when coming in, for instance, one may breathe in slowly as they count to four and breathe out even slower as they count to eight.

This slow, deep, and deliberate breathing will help relax your breath and return into a normal, relaxed state. Since all things present in the body are interconnected, controlling, and relaxing one's breath should in turn control and relax muscle tensions that are caused by anger thereby reducing feelings of anger significantly.

Progressive Muscle Relaxation

One of the other noticeable physical changes related to anger is muscle tension. This tension can manifest in different parts of one's body and can collectively clump in specific areas such as the neck and shoulders. This tension can even remain long after the anger is gone. Progressive muscle relaxation involves deliberately tensing and tightening your muscles both stressed and unstressed for a slow count of ten then relaxing or releasing these tightened muscles. When practicing this, be sure to release muscles immediately you feel pain. This technique requires you to work progressively from one muscle group to another (for example from head to toe) until you have taken each muscle through a cycle of tension and release. With diligent practice, one may notice their ability to do this cycle of the full body in a few minutes. This technique of tightening and releasing muscles can prove more relaxing than relaxation itself.

Visualizing Yourself to Calmness

Visualization refers to the mental formation or representation of an object, image, situation or set of information. Visualization techniques can also be employed to help with the management of anger. Our brains constantly visualize in the process of simulating future scenarios. This visualization happens so effortlessly that we barely notice it in the same way we barely notice our breathing. When we become aware of our visualization, we can use it as a tool to reduce or reverse anger. Visualization to help with anger is done by imagining a place or scenario that makes you feel calm or relaxed and focusing on details (sometimes with the aid of audio material such as music) such as smells, sounds and how good it feels to be in that space. This is usually done when one is sited comfortably and quietly with their eyes closed.

Visualization has four key benefits that improve how we deal with anger. Firstly, it rewires and programs one's brain to help them realize the strategies, tools, and resources they can use to achieve peace and harmony away from anger. Secondly, it builds our intrinsic motivation to take actions necessary to change the habit pattern of the mind, which is reacting to anger. Thirdly, it sparks one's creative subconscious, which helps us with the sublimation of these negative feelings into more socially acceptable forms of expression such as dance, poetry, music among others. This sublimation helps us express rather than suppress these feelings of anger. Lastly, visualization aids in the law of attraction thereby drawing you closer to circumstances, resources, tools, and people who can help you achieve your goals of anger management.

Various meditation techniques are also used in anger management and relaxation. Mindfulness meditation and Vipassana meditation both encourage us to accept the anger when it manifests itself and observe it as it is without reacting to it or engaging with it. This usually causes us to be fueled and consumed by it causing it to become problematic. In retrospect, when we just simply observe anger as an emotion, neither good nor bad, we learn to work with anger, as it is however or whenever it arises skillfully without it spiraling out of control. When we engage in guided meditation we learn how to relax and gain relief from stress and stressors that may end up causing anger and allow us to process these feelings healthily. This technique can be used with children too especially those with heavy temper tantrums. Peaceful and guided meditations help children, adults, and teens improve self-esteem, relieve anxiety, and stress, and feel generally refreshed in mind, body, and spirit and develop positive mental attitudes in their daily activities.

Grief Management

Grief can be defined as the heightened sense or feeling of pain we feel when we experience loss. This pain is severe as the loss is a reflection of something or someone we love and one may feel engulfed and overwhelmed by it. Grief can follow the loss of someone such as the death of a loved one or the destruction of a relationship to the loss of a pet or even something like the loss of your home. Grief is complex and has no specific rules or set timing. Grief can have symptoms similar to depression such as insomnia, sadness, and loss of interest in self-care. Grief is different from depression as it doesn't impair self-worth. However, grief is not experienced by everyone in the same way. In some cases, it may be accompanied by feelings of guilt or confusion. Prolonged grief can last up to months if not dealt with and can result in isolation as well as chronic loneliness. Nevertheless, its symptoms tend to lessen over time but can be triggered by anniversaries or thoughts about the loss at whatever time.

It has been proposed by professionals in psychology that grief has five stages. These are denial, anger, bargaining, depression, and acceptance. Denial is the first stage of grief and is characterized by the world feeling overwhelming and meaningless. We tend to feel numb and as though life makes absolutely no sense and we wonder how we can go on. In the case of the loss of a loved one, for instance, one may be thinking they cannot live without the deceased and wondering what the point to life without them is. The next stage of grief, which is essential for the healing process, is anger. In the same case, one may be asking questions like "Why did they have to die so soon?" or "Where is God in all of this?"

As one progresses on the path of grief, they get to the next stage of bargaining where one feels like they would do and sacrifice anything and everything for their loved one to be spared their demise. In this case one may begin praying and making promissory offerings to their particular God or Goddess saying things like "I promise to be a better child to my parent if you bring them back," or "I promise to do better for the community if I wake up from this and it's just a dream." During this stage, one is engulfed in 'what-ifs' and 'if only's'. After bargaining, we tend to go deeper into the grief as we bring our attention to the present and face the feelings of emptiness and sadness caused by our loss. This stage usually and feels everlasting, however, it is important to understand that it is an appropriate response to great loss and it will not last forever. This is not a clinical depression or a sign of mental illness.

The last stage of acceptance is usually mixed up with the idea that we should be okay with the loss. However, in reality, most people are never okay with the loss they experience. We usually just learn how to live with it accepting the reality as it is and not as we would like it to be. We accept the new reality as the permanent reality and making it the norm, which we have to adjust to and learn to live with.

Without a doubt, grief is related to and can cause or be caused by stress. Change is one of the reasons stress and grief are intertwined when you lose something, you have to reboot and rearrange things about your life that were connected to the loss, which can potentially act as a stressor. Another reason for this relationship is the pressure from yourself and sometimes society to get over your loss, move on and become 'normal' again. Interpersonal stressors such as hurt feelings, conflict and feelings of alienation and isolation from family and friends following the loss of someone can also be related to this relationship between grief and stress. Internal conflict and an overload of emotions which one usually feel unequipped to handle is another reason for this relationship. Lastly, frustrations that come from not getting what you want are another connecting factor to this relationship. When one experiences grief and loss, they tend to want back what they have lost or wanted a change in circumstances, but our wishes are not what we have in reality causing frustration and stress.

How to Meditate for Grief and Loss

Meditation for grief is one of the most effective ways to deal with grief and loss by helping us get rid of the symptoms of depression and anxiety, pain as well as mend our relationships with others and bring us closure through introspection and reorientation. Breathing meditation and relaxing meditation techniques are good to restore a state of calmness in the mind and body as well as help alleviate certain pains. Guided meditations help us reduce the suffering that comes together with grief. According to teachers of these guided meditations such as Shinzen Young, suffering is a result of pain and resistance. With this understanding, one realizes that they should not resist the loss that has already happened and that they should accept it as part of the experiences in their lives. In as much as pain could be harder to eradicate as it is the mark and relic of love, this understanding reduces suffering significantly and gives us a boost to work patiently and mindfully with ourselves as we reengage with life after whatever loss you have gone through. Mindfulness meditations as well as Vipassana meditation work in this same manner aiming to eradicate the suffering that is accompanied by grief.

Chapter 14
Stress and Workplace Awareness Meditation

When working somewhere, one is usually in a different environment with people from all walks of life and pressures from authority figures and oneself. These objects and situations can potentially be acute stressors and trigger; therefore, the stress in the workplace is normal. However, when stress becomes extreme and overwhelming, it can interfere with your productivity, relationships with colleagues, performance, mental and physical health and also spill out to other aspects of your life such as your relationships with friends and family.

While one cannot control the entire workplace environment, there is no need to feel defeated when faced with a difficult situation that triggers stress. When faced with stressors, some steps can be taken to improve your coping skills, relationships in and out of work, productivity, job satisfaction and overall well-being no matter what your individual goals, work demands, and ambitions may be.

Meditation is among the best practices to come out of stressful situations especially at work almost immediately. It works by helping us to regulate our emotions and retuning the brain to be more resilient to stressors. Practicing meditation in the workplace increases our productivity and motivation by turning stress into success. Most people may think of meditation as another task on their to-do list with the demands of a quiet and calm place; however, it is important to understand and take meditation as being able to be in the midst of trouble, noise, and hard work while maintaining calmness and equanimity in your heart. The two most recommended forms of meditation to manage stress in the workplace are transcendental meditation and mindfulness meditation.

Transcendental meditation has a great deal of research backing its ability to help relieve stress at the workplace and reduce cortisol and anxiety. Continuous and diligent practice of transcendental meditation shows to notably improve productivity and work satisfaction so much that business owners and large companies such as General Motors, Sony, Toyota, and IBM are beginning to invest in meditation programs and making them available for their employees to double their output and wellbeing. This form of meditation shows to improve emotional intelligence, which in turn advances the relationships you have with your colleagues and helps you effectively deal with and express your own emotions.

Mindfulness meditation as a way to deal with workplace stress is more commonly practiced due to the rise in popularity of the practice over the last few years. This technique aims to improve our clarity in our worldly perceptions, which consequently helps us make better decisions. Moreover, being less agitated results in greater inner strength and more stable emotions leading us to be happier and have more fulfilling lives. To reap these benefits, it is important to start meditating especially at the beginning of your day or before you begin working. This can be even easier if you start a meditation group at work with some colleagues and practice mindfulness meditation together before you begin working. It is important to also practice mindful breathing where you randomly take 3-5 mindful breaths and go back to doing what you were doing.

In addition to this, it is also essential to take advantage of the time you use walking as an opportunity to meditate and practice mindful walking. Here one observes their walking with deep awareness and if not in a hurry, it would not hurt to slow down and let your mind follow. Another essential practice tied to mindfulness meditation in the workplace is deep listening. In this case, one listens wholesomely with the intent of understanding as opposed to replying. Normally when we listen with the intent to reply we are usually thinking about our next statement and how to interject our particular opinion rather than taking time to pay attention to and understand fully what the other party has to say. This practice will improve workplace relationships and reduce the frictions and arguments that cause stress at work. Lastly, the practice of mindful speech will also help reduce stress by improving our overall interactions and relationships. When speaking mindfully, one takes the time to think about what they are about to say and visualize and understand the impact it will have on the recipient of the message whether positive or negative. In this case, it is important to consider how our statements will be interpreted and try our best to convey information that will elicit positive consequences and responses.

Abdominal Breathing for Impulse Control

Occasional impulsive behavior is a normal part of life. We experience and engage in impulsivity from time to time whether it is by eating a slice of pizza when on a diet or buying something we do not need. For a person without impulse control however, it is difficult to resist sudden urges, which more often than not seem forceful. For such individuals, it seems like activities that would be deemed normal if done less frequently or less intensely are out of their control. Many are the occasions that these impulsive behaviors violate other people's rights and cause conflict with whatever societal values and norms put in place by one's culture or society. These impulses tend to occur frequently and rapidly without the consideration of the consequences it may breed.

A problem with impulse control is usually noted by a constant repetition of the behavior despite negative consequences, experiencing strong cravings and urges to engage in the problematic behavior, incapability to have power over problem behaviors and engaging in problem behavior to feel pleasure or relieve pressure. Some other symptoms of impulse control are obsessive thoughts, inability to delay instant gratification, lack of patience and severe tension and/or anxiety experienced before engaging in the impulsive behavior. Impulse control can be a key feature or symptom in some mental illnesses such as bulimia and paraphilia; however, some types of impulse control disorders stand as disorders by themselves. Some of the most common forms of impulse control disorders are:

- **Pyromania**   this is the inability to control the urge to set fires. A person with pyromania usually reports feelings for pleasure following their behavior or relief from anxiety or emotional blockage.

- **Kleptomania**   this refers to the uncontrollable urge to steal something and is different from stealing for a necessity such as water or food. In this case, people steal things that are meaningless and unnecessary.

- **Trichotillomania**   This is a disorder that is usually characterized by a strong urge to pull out ones hair. Even when this act is painful, the urge surpasses any concern for pain.

- **Intermittent explosive disorder**   this refers to the inability to control anger outbursts to even the smallest of triggers whereby the rage can spill out of control and turn into physical acts of violence.

- **Pathological gambling**   also referred to as compulsive gambling it was once considered an impulse control disorder but recent research shows that it is more of a process addiction. Here one is unable to resist the urge to gamble. The thought of gambling becomes too overpowering causing one to feel like engaging in gambling is the only relief they can get.

- **Unspecified impulse-control disorder**   in this case, one shows the general signs and symptoms of an impulse-control disorder however, the impulse observed does not fall into any pre-recognized criteria.

One of the most recommended techniques to control one's impulses is abdominal breathing. This technique is similar to mindful breathing in that one deliberately slows down and deepens their breath. When practicing this, you need to inhale slowly through your nose then exhale even slower through your mouth while making a hissing sound almost like a balloon losing air trying to make the hiss last as long as possible. This technique involves controlling your breath to calm you down and reduce your cravings and urges.

Chapter 15
Meditative Guide For Positive Consciousness

As one of the simplest forms of meditation, positive consciousness works almost exclusively on the rebuilding of conscious mind maps. For whatever reason, at some point in your life, your self-esteem, your self-confidence, and your courage to move forward have all been tampered with.

By focusing on positive consciousness, you can attempt to see all these self-inflicted wounds. No longer are your thoughts at the mercy of other people's perceptions of you. In contrast, you will now become whoever it is that you need to be in order to meet your own demands and aspirations. As you seek a suitable position to begin this meditation, stretch out your body to first rid it of any wasteful energy that has been left over from the day before.

As you seat yourself, stretch out your back until you feel a sharp pull, and at this point, lower your neck to be level with the floor. Outstretch your arms upon the tops of your knees and lift your palms upward and leave them facing toward you.

You are now ready to start your meditative guide.

As you slowly close your eyes, fix within your mind's eye a point from which you are meant to gather all consciousness.

Remember that your consciousness has suffered in recent days and, as such, is in need of healing. By promoting positive consciousness, not only are you rebuilding this broken stream of good will, but you are fortifying it so that it will be protected from any future harm.

Breathe in carefully to the count of five.

Hold to the count of four and then slowly release.

You are resilient.

You are calm.

You are undisturbed.

You are gifted.

Exhale deeply, purging yourself of all the negative stress and energy that has been building in your body, and instead, open your mind's eye and with it, you should be able to see and feel the energies around you.

You are seeking within yourself a way in which you can let go and be at peace.

The cool darkness behind your eyes is inviting you to feel calm and at peace. The bright lights at the periphery of your mind are showing you the endless possibilities that you have at your disposal.

I am capable.

I am smart.

I am efficient.

I am worthy.

I am talented.

I am resourceful.

I am bright.

I am attentive.

As you remind yourself of these things, open your mind once again to see the various energies that are flowing through your being. With your mind, start to follow each individual channel of energy until you can see how they flow beautifully into each other.

This time, as you repeat each positive affirmation, weave it through one of the strands of energy so that it will flow perfectly though your mind from now on and forever after.

I am capable.

I am smart.

I am efficient.

I am worthy.

I am talented.

I am resourceful.

I am bright.

I am attentive.

Each of these thoughts is now an inviolable part of your consciousness. As your energy begins to build in your center, allow it to move upward to your mind and, as you raise your neck, lift your face forward to accept the new revolutionary truths that have become a part of your reality.

You are powerful.

You are significant.

You are respected.

You are loved.

Repeat the last four phrases in your mind once again.

I am powerful.

I am significant.

I am respected.

I am loved.

Breathe in.

Release.

Breathe in.

Release.

Breathe in.

Release.

As you prepare yourself to open your eyes, you are embodying a positively minded individual.

Chapter 16
Daily Meditation Affirmation Routines

Morning Affirmations Meditation

Are you looking to start off your day on the right side of the bed? If you want to wake up energetic and ready for any day ahead of you, I highly suggest starting your day off with a morning meditation, topped off with some positive affirmations to get you in a positive mindset.

Of course, you can listen to this meditation at any time of the day, but it is a perfect start to your morning and will only take a small amount of time to energize you and get you started!

As we start this meditation, I now invite you to go ahead and take some deep breaths. With each breath you take, allow the airflow to begin to energize you. Inhale deep into your lungs and exhale everything out.

Breathe in...and exhale. Allow for your breaths to be slow, deep, and calm. Each breath you take brings in the air that your body needs to help get you started. Allow your breaths to fill you with energy and let go of any fatigue you may be feeling at this moment. For the next few moments, this is all I want you to focus on. Just concentrate on your breath. It does not matter what tasks you have for the rest of the day. All you need to think about is breathing in, breathing out, and getting your energy set up for the day.

[Pause]

You are going to be ready for this day ahead of you. Breathe in positive energy and allow all positive thoughts to enter your mind. With your next few exhales, let any negative feelings go. If you feel any tension built up in your body, let that go too. You do not have the time nor the energy to waste on negativity. There is only energy and positivity right now. Breathe and remind yourself to be positive.

[Pause]

Now, I want you to squeeze your hands into fists gently. As you do this, feel as the muscles strengthen in your arms and your shoulders. Feel now as the strength and energy begin to flow through your veins. You are powerful, and you can accomplish anything you want to. You are capable of accomplishing anything that you need to get done today. You can do anything you put your mind to. Now, relax your fists, and allow your muscles to relax.

[Pause]

As your body begins to awaken, feel how warm and energetic you are starting to feel. If you would like, try to open and close your hands a few times. I want you to become mindful of how wonderful your body feels as it wakes up, ready to tackle anything that comes at you today. Allow yourself to become excited for the day, ready for anything that can happen today; there are so many possibilities. Feel now as this positive energy waves through your body and allow your mind and soul to become alive.

[Pause]

If you are feeling up to it, I now invite you to enjoy a gentle stretch to get your muscles going. Go ahead and place your fingertips together and gently stretch your arms above your head. Reach for the ceiling and feel the soft pull down your shoulders and into your sides. If you want, gently lean from side to side and feel as your muscles begin to warm up. When you are ready, bring your arms back down and bring your awareness to your toes. Take a deep breath and allow the energy to surge through you.

[Pause]

Next, I want you to start to wiggle your feet a little. As you flex your feet, feel as the muscles in your legs enjoy a gentle stretch. Go ahead and spend some time waking your legs up. They are well rested from the night before and are ready to be put to work! Now, hold your feet still and enjoy the sensation of energy tingling through your toes, into your ankles, and up your legs. Take another deep breath in and allow for these sensations to wash over your whole body. The more you move, the more energetic you begin to feel.

[Pause]

Now that your body is awake and feeling energetic, it is time to open your mind to positive thoughts to carry you through the day. In the next few moments, we will go over some self-esteem affirmations to boost your confidence and get you excited for the day ahead of you. If, at any point in your day, you feel your stress and anxiety start to take over, I invite you to take a few moments to breathe and repeat the following affirmations to yourself.

As I say the following affirmations, I invite you to continue to focus on your breathing and stretch; however, you feel fit. If you still feel tense in some areas, go ahead and stretch these areas out. This is your time; use it to your advantage.

If you start your day off on a positive note, it can get better from there, even if you hit a couple of rocky patches. Feel free to repeat after me or simply listen to the following; it is completely up to you.

I am capable of achieving anything that I work hard for.

[Pause]

When times get tough, I have the ability to work through them.

[Pause]

I deserve to be happy.

[Pause]

I am a strong individual, and I am in charge of my life, even when I cannot control the circumstances.

[Pause]

I am worthwhile, even when people make me feel like I am not.

[Pause]

I accept myself for who I am.

[Pause]

I am proud of all of my hard work and accomplishments.

[Pause]

I deserve happiness because I work hard for it.

[Pause]

I have many wonderful qualities.

[Pause]

I love myself.

[Pause]

I am grateful for my life.

[Pause]

I am grateful for all of this energy I am feeling.

[Pause]

I am ready to tackle this day and anything that comes my way.

[Pause]

I will handle everything with as much grace as possible.

[Pause]

In tough times, I will remember to breathe and remain calm.

[Pause]

I am in control of my thoughts and my body.

[Pause]

I choose to be calm and peaceful throughout the day.

[Pause]

I am ready to get started with this day and will remember to be at peace.

[Pause]

Fantastic. As we draw this meditation to a close, take a few more moments to breathe on your own time and focus your thoughts and intentions for the day. When things become overwhelming, remember to find your breath, and you can work through just about anything. At the end of the day, it all comes down to your mindset, and by starting with this meditation, you are ready to overcome anything with positivity. Now, breathe and get ready to start your day.

[Pause]

Meditation Time: 40 Minutes

Breathing Awareness Meditation

Before we begin this meditation, I now invite you to find a position that is comfortable for you. As you settle in, take a few moments to make sure all distractions such as your cellphone and laptop are closed. For the next few minutes, I would like you to just focus on yourself. As you meditate, there is nothing else that matters. If you are feeling anxious right now, that is perfectly okay. We all go through these feelings. What matters right now is that you do something about it.

[Pause]

As you settle into position, go ahead and take a nice, deep breath in. If you would like, allow for your eyes to begin to flutter closed. If you are not comfortable with this, simply keep them open and start to soften your gaze. When you are comfortable, all I would like you to do is find your breath. With each breath you take, simply become mindful of how it feels to breathe in fully and exhale everything out. When we feel anxious, we often forget the very basic concept of breathing. Our thoughts begin to move quickly, and our breathing patterns begin to match. Perhaps you are mindful of this, but most likely, you had no idea because you were so focused on being anxious, and that is okay! Just breathe and tune your focus in on yourself.

[Pause]

Right now, all you need to focus on is the air entering through your nostrils. It does not matter why you feel anxious, and it does not matter what tasks need to be completed once this meditation is finished. Allow for all of the thoughts in your head to exit and focus only on your breath.

[Pause]

On your next breath, I want you to become mindful of how the air travels into your lungs and allow for your belly to expand fully. As you breathe out, feel how your belly gets smaller, and the air moves peacefully back out through your mouth or nose. You may notice that you inhale, feels different from your exhale. Breathe in and feel the comfort of the cool air as it enters your body and how warm it feels as it leaves.

[Pause]

If you ever become distracted during your practice, that is perfectly okay. We all get distracted sometimes. If you find yourself getting distracted by noise or thoughts, allow these to pass without judgment and bring your focus back in yourself. There is no need to change anything right now. All you are doing is relaxing and breathing. Simply bring your attention back to your breath and continue a few more moments to breathe on your own.

[Pause]

If you would like, you can count with me as you continue to find your breath. On your next breath, I invite you to hold the breath for a few beats. Allow for the air in your lungs to nourish your body and your thoughts. I want each breath to relax you and clear your mind of all worry. When you are ready, we can begin.

Breathe in softly...and hold for one...two...three...and slowly release. Excellent.

Let's do that two more times together.

Breathe in softly...and hold for one...two...three...and release.

[Pause]

Breathe in...and hold for one...two...three...and slowly release.

[Pause]

Wonderful. At this point, you are probably already feeling much better. Go ahead and take a few more breaths on your own time.

[Pause]

During times of anxiety, I want this to be the first practice that pops into your mind. While breathing is a simple task, it can be highly effective. We all experience anxiety in different ways. If you start to become overwhelmed with tasks or emotions, take a step back and find your breath. With each breath you take, gently remind yourself that these feelings will pass, and as long as you are breathing, you are going to be okay. When you are ready, we can continue to the next meditation to keep working through overcoming your anxiety.

Meditation Time: 15 Minutes

The 3 Minutes Breathing Space

This simple exercise is utilized in MBCT programs and Cognitive Behavior Therapies. It helps people get unstuck and move forward with their lives, even after embarrassing breakdowns.

While performing this mindfulness practice, refrain from evaluating and choosing your thoughts. Instead, you have to become aware of them and your breathing. The previous exercises made you concentrate on one part of your body.

Contrastingly, the 3 minutes breathing space will make you expand your senses. As a beginner, you will only be required to focus on your breathing. But you have to be mindful of the effect of respiration on various areas of your body. Feel the sensations it creates and its effects on your body as a whole.

Does that sound too complicated? Well, don't fret because it is very easy to practice. It only involves 3 simple steps.

a) Firstly, look for a comfortable area wherein you can't be disturbed by anyone. And if possible, turn off your cellphone and laptop. There must be no distractions. Next, notice the thoughts inside your head, and don't change the things you're observing.

b) The second step involves focusing on your breathing. Sit in a covered flat surface and sit up straight. Once you are settled, concentrate on your intake and expelling of air. Be aware of the rise and fall of your chest and abdomen. Feel the air as it enters and escapes your nostrils. What do you smell? Do you hear your breathing?

c) Third, you have to expand your senses. You should still focus on your breathing, but all the while, you must be aware of the other sensations your body is feeling. Other noise or disturbances are unnecessary. Are your legs cramping? Do you feel hot or cold? Be aware and focus on those sensations as well.

The goal of this exercise is to establish awareness for body sensations and to emphasize shifting of attention and to move on from one focus to another. Accordingly, you should only linger for a minute in each step. The 3MBS exercise prepares you for other mindfulness practices, and it encourages "moving of attention."

The exercise can help you get unstuck from automatic routines. It also provides you space wherein you can get a breather from stress or taxing tasks.

Mindfulness on the Bus or Train

If you utilize public transportation, you can take the time spent getting where you are going to practice mindfulness meditation as effectively as if you were sequestered peacefully in your own home. There is one caveat; however, in order to practice mindfulness meditation effectively, it is important that you feel comfortable in the space in which you find yourself. If you find yourself in a situation where something requires your full attention, you will likely be unable to reach your full mindfulness meditation potential.

While listening to music while practicing mindfulness meditation in public is not recommended, you may find it helpful to wear headphones as this is a clear signal to those around you that you do not wish to be disturbed. Furthermore, you may find it helpful to set some type of timer because when you get into the zone while being mindful, it can be easy to lose track of time.

With the preliminaries out of the way, the first thing that you are going to want to do is to plant your feet firmly a comfortable distance apart from one another, whether you are standing or sitting. If standing, take care that you are in a place where you can easily keep your balance. With your feet firmly planted, slowly stretch out your body so that you assume the proper posture for your current surroundings. Take a moment to feel your body move with the rhythm of the train/bus and consider how you are connected not just to the transportation you are riding but to all of those who are sharing the journey with you.

Once you feel that you are centered, choose a spot in front of you that is approximately three feet from your current position. Choose a spot that is close to the ground, perhaps just a foot or two above the floor of the bus or train. Slowly lower your eyes to this point on the ground without lowering your neck, it is important to maintain proper posture throughout the exercise. As you feel your eyes begin to dip towards the floor, focus exclusively on all of the sensory information they are providing you. From there, slowly incorporate the sensations that are being provided by the rest of your senses.

In order to tune out all of the noise and movement that naturally comes with riding public transportation, focus on your breathing and concentrate on taking deep rhythmic breaths at a nice slow pace. Once you have found a rhythm that works for you, consider one of the options below as a means of focusing your attention and attaining a state of mindfulness that might not seem possible otherwise. Remember, practicing mindfulness meditation while using public transportation is even trickier to get the hang of than the other types of mindfulness meditation in these pages. Don't get discouraged if you can't clear your mind as easily as you may be able to elsewhere, as with any other skill practice makes perfect.

Chapter 17
Affirmations For Over Coming Anxiety

Anxiety, as you have learned thus far, is something that is largely pervasive, annoying, something people wish they had less of but is entirely common. Many people suffer from anxiety, and in recognizing that fact, you are better able to feel less ashamed. Do not be ashamed of your anxiety— so many people around you probably share some of your same anxiety symptoms and you would never realize it. Nevertheless, it is something that you should make an effort to correct. As you master these methods, learning to create affirmations and learning to fake it until you make it, you will be able to get a better hold on any symptoms that arise for you.

Creating Affirmations

Affirmations are short sentences that you tell yourself in order to serve as a reminder or as a replacement for a negative thought. They are easy to use and are most often used as a quick and easy repetition in order to overcome negative thinking. You can use them specifically for anxiety, but they can also be used for general mood regulation, encouraging good habits, and many other situations in your life that require more self-discipline.

Your affirmation can be anything, so long as you ensure that it follows the right structure—it must be present, positive, and personal. By ensuring these three things, you are able to make an affirmation that is largely functional simply because you will be able to control it.

When you ensure that your affirmation is positive, you are respecting the cycle between thoughts, feelings, and behaviors. You know that a positive thought will lead to positive feelings, which will lead to positive behaviors, which is what you are hoping to achieve with your positive affirmation. After all, any affirmation you are developing is meant to help you cope with anxiety, which is largely comprised of negative thinking in the first place. The reason it must be positive can be clearly understood with the following example: Consider two affirmations and decide which seems more motivational or helpful for your anxiety:

I will not let my anxiety control me

I control my anxiety by remembering my breathing techniques

Chances are, you would find the second statement more useful in controlling your anxiety. This is for a very good reason—you are creating an action for yourself instead of telling yourself what not to do. When you know what not to do, you still do not know what you should be doing, after all. You will be unsure whether what you should be doing is crying, letting anger take control, or even just abandoning ship altogether. You do not have a clear action. However, when you tell yourself that you will control anxiety through breathing techniques, you remind yourself that you have a method to ensure that things are okay and you have an action plan for when anxiety starts to rise.

Next, you must make sure that your affirmation is present-tense. The reason for this is that you want to ensure that your affirmation is currently true. By creating an affirmation that is present-tense and repeating it to yourself, you tell yourself that it is currently true at that moment, which can sometimes be enough to trigger the behavior you needed to see. You are able to essentially trick your brain into action by saying that you are engaging in whatever behavior your affirmation is asking for.

When you make your affirmation something future tense by saying something like, "I will control my anxiety," you do not tell yourself when it will happen. It could happen tomorrow, it could happen a year for now, or it could happen right that moment, but it is ambiguous. Remember, part of anxiety is a concern about uncertainty, and ambiguity absolutely breeds uncertainty.

Lastly, your affirmation must be personal. Remember what self-discipline taught you—only you can control yourself, and you can only control yourself. Keep in mind that those are two different things altogether, though they look like someone was distracted when writing—the only one who can make you do anything is yourself, and the only thing you have utter control over is yourself. Because of that, the only way you can ensure your affirmation is true is through making sure that it is personal. You want to be the subject that is doing whatever action is in your affirmation in order to make sure that you can absolutely guarantee that the affirmation will be true. For example, you could say, "Jill will control anxiety through breathing," but you cannot enforce that. You can, however, enforce, "I am encouraging Jill to control her anxiety through breathing." Now, your affirmation focuses on something you can control.

Some examples of anxiety-related affirmations can include:

- I am safe where I am right now

- I control my actions, even when I am anxious

- I have everything I need to control my anxiety

- I use my breathing to keep myself under my own control

Notice how each and every one of those examples starts with "I," involves some sort of statement, and is present tense. Those are perfect examples. You can create any sort of affirmation for yourself, so long as it matches that pattern.

When you are using affirmations, you want to use them with plenty of repetition. You will be repeating them to yourself regularly, and because of that, you want to develop some sort of routine for yourself. For example, pair your affirmation reciting with some other activity that you do regularly. You may decide to pair it with getting into your car as you buckle up. When you match up your repetition of affirmations with an activity that you do regularly or automatically already, you can then make that affirmation just as habitual.

If you choose to get into the car and buckling up as your example, every time you do, you will recite your affirmation to yourself at least 10 times as you do. It does not matter how many times you get in and out of your car—you will repeat those affirmations. If you happen to get in your car at least 10 times, then you are reciting those affirmations at least 100 times that day. Do not worry though—the more repetition you implement the better. Over time, the thoughts become habitual and will happen without you thinking about them. That is how you know it is working and that your mind is accepting them as true.

As you make them true for yourself, you will have to also correct yourself every time you come close to making your affirmation not true as well— for example, if you are going to lose control of yourself, you should recite your affirmation to you. Your affirmation is a sort of back-up plan, reminding you of what to do in that particular situation and by reminding yourself, you are able to better gain control over the situation at hand. If you are close to losing control of your anxiety and recite the affirmation, you remind yourself that you can, in fact, control it, and you trigger your breathing exercises. If you feel like you are going to lose your temper, you can recite your affirmation related to that and feel the desire to lash out fade away.

Fake it until You Make it

When you are struggling to get that anxiety under control, sometimes, the best solution is to actually fake that you are in better control of it. Some of the techniques you have already studied already introduced this topic—when you engaged in the breathing and relaxation techniques, you were forcing your brain to accept a state that it was not naturally in. You essentially fooled it into thinking that you were calmer than you actually were just because you changed your pace in breathing. Much of your body behaves like this, and you can actually change a lot of your own feelings just by acting the part. Even if you do not feel confident right at that moment, you will the more you practice it.

Anxiety is particularly tricky in the sense that not only does it trigger certain feelings from you, but it is also triggered by certain physical states. This makes it essentially self-fulfilling—it can encourage the feelings that add fuel to the fire, making it easily escalated, and therefore destructive if left unchecked. However, when you instead begin to respond to your anxiety in ways that are not anxious, the anxiety starts to melt away.

Stop and think about what you would not do during an emergency—you would probably not remain calm as you spoke or smile. You would not be relaxed or eating or breathing slowly. You would not have a relaxed body posture. You would not relax back in your chair. All of those would not match an actual emergency that would require action.

When you behave in any of those ways when you are anxious, even if you only choose one of those behaviors, you are able to tell your mind that there is no real threat. If there were a threat, you tell your mind, then you would not be talking calmly or resting. You would not be breathing deeply and calmly. If there were an actual threat to yourself at that moment, you would be panicking, running away, or otherwise attempting to escape something that is not actually there at that moment in time.

One way to trigger this is by keeping candy or gum on your person at all times. When you begin to feel anxious, you can stop, take out that candy or gum, and put it in your mouth. Think about it this way—if you were actually in danger, or you were actually in an emergency, would you have the time to stop, pull out a stick of gum, open it, put away the wrapper, put the packaging away, and put the gum in your mouth to chew? No, probably not—you would be focusing on survival or helping someone else to survive. You would not be able to salivate if you were under threat, but even though you are feeling anxious at that moment, you are able to salivate with the gum in your mouth. That contradiction triggers your brain to stop, reevaluate, and instead switch to calmness rather than focusing on the negative or the fear associated with whatever you are doing at that particular moment.

Because anxiety has a tendency to be about what will come next, you are able to trick yourself, telling yourself that what will come next is not a debilitating disaster, but rather some sort of sweet treat instead. Your body will quickly cease the fear and anxiety and shift instead to something more relaxed.

Conclusion

If you have gotten to this point it is because you are committed to learning about the ways in which meditation can have a profoundly positive effect in your life.

As such, the next step is to put what you have learned into practice. That is, from the reduction of stress, anxiety, insomnia and even pain, the benefits of meditations somewhat keep mocking its naysayers. The more research conducted, the more the previous sentence makes sense. Thousands of research reports continue to prove how meditation influences both the mental and physical wellbeing. Meditation can bridge the gap between you and many worldly wants as well: your sleep gets better, you are able to regulate your weight, your relationships become more satisfactory and you have the ability to reduce physical pains that occasionally come and go.

Although its practice is still being blindsided by many factors, the practice is bound to receive the recognition it deserves eventually. With the internet of things, the spread of the practice is almost reaching a rampant state with the topic of meditation resting on the lips of both professionals and paupers. Even in the event that most of these people are just talking about it without putting any practice, the fact that it has gained such a massive amount of popularity is nothing but astounding. This is a positive thing though, as the positives of meditation outweigh the negatives.

For those who are a bit skeptical about engaging in it because of various reasons, I hope this book serves as a beacon of light to dispel any misbeliefs and doubts one might carry about the practice. The main purpose of meditation is to reach within and access oneself. We all spend so much time on a daily basis trying to find people and things. It all falls in place easier if you discover the most important thing to find is yourself.

So, thank you once again for your kind attention. If you have found this book to be useful or helpful, in any way, please tell your friends and family, or anyone whom you believe to be interested in this topic, about this book. It will surely help them find the balance they seek in life. In addition, they are surely going to benefit in the long run.

CPSIA information can be obtained
at www.ICGtesting.com
Printed in the USA
LVHW020448120221
679113LV00010B/269

9 781801 690447